THE SILENT FALL

*A Secret Service Agent's Story
of Tragedy and Triumph after 9/11*

SAMANTHA HORWITZ

© 2016 Courage To Win, LLC. All rights reserved. No part of this book may be reproduced, scanned, or distributed in any printed or electronic form without permission.

Note: Some names and identifying details have been changed to protect the privacy of individuals.

Cover: Original design and artwork by David Snider. Original cover concept by Lee Aks and Dustin Semmig.

Interior: Claudia Volkman

ISBN: 978-0-9978026-0-3 (soft cover)
ISBN: 978-0-9978026-1-0 (e-book)

Printed in the United States of America

5 4 3 2 1

This book is dedicated to the brave men and women in blue, red, and green who courageously put their lives on the line every day, and to those who paid the ultimate price so we may enjoy our freedom.

10/15/16

To Jim

BE COURAGEOUS!

TABLE OF CONTENTS

Survival—A Family Trait   7

PART ONE: TRAGEDY

One—Just Another Day at the Office   11

Two—Heading Home   27

Three—The New Normal   45

Four—The Debriefing   59

Five—Warning Signs   75

Six—Back to Work   93

PART TWO: FROM TRAUMA TO TRIUMPH

Seven—A Rocky Start   107

Eight—Reality Check   123

Nine—New Beginnings   135

Ten—The Answer   157

Eleven—Lessons for Life   173

Epilogue   185

Acknowledgments   191

About the Author   195

SURVIVAL—A FAMILY TRAIT

It is not the strongest or the most intelligent who will survive but those who can best manage change.
—Leon C. Megginson

April 15, 1912
A baby and his mother file onto the deck of the RMS Titanic, ready to be lowered into a lifeboat. Unexpectedly, from behind, the baby is knocked from his mother's arms and miraculously lands in the lap of a woman sitting in a lifeboat several decks below.

Hours later, aboard the RMS Carpathia, the distraught mother who thought her baby was lost forever hears a familiar cry. She turns to see her son in the arms of a stranger. She rushes over to the woman, who claims the baby as her own. Captain Rostron, the captain of the RMS Carpathia, is summoned to solve the dispute. Who does the baby belong to?

One story says that the baby was identified by a strawberry birthmark on his chest (see Encyclopedia-Titanica.org). The family story—the *real* story—is that the baby was identified by the fact that he was circumcised, a practice performed on Jewish male babies. The woman holding the baby in her arms aboard the Carpathia was of Italian decent, not Jewish. It was not difficult for Captain Rostron to return the baby to his rightful mother. Why the discrepancy in stories? In 1912 the word *circumcision* was not one mentioned in public.

This is the story of my Great Uncle Phil "Filly" Aks and his mother, my great-grandmother, Leah Aks.

August 8, 1942
The USS George F. Elliott is in the Pacific Ocean, transporting the United States Marines to the amphibious assault on Guadalcanal. A young Navy lieutenant commander is on the deck of the ship having a conversation with a fellow soldier. Out of nowhere, Japanese planes appear. He looks up to see a plane flying right at him. There is a huge explosion—the soldier he was talking with moments before is gone. Minutes later he finds himself in the water, his face burning. The USS George F. Elliot sinks into the Pacific.

The young man goes on to become one of the most successful dentists in Virginia. The impact of the battle has such a profound effect on him that he names his oldest daughter after his ship.

This is the story of my grandfather, Harry Aks. His daughter, Victoria Elliot Aks, is my mom.

September 11, 2001
In my wildest dreams I never expected to be added to the list of family members who would make history—and SURVIVE.

This is my story . . .

PART ONE
TRAGEDY

ONE

JUST ANOTHER DAY AT THE OFFICE

SEPTEMBER 11, 2001, was a day like any other day: Up early, work out, shower, and off to work. It seemed like the faster I tried to go, the more traffic worked against me until I was stopped completely on the Newark Bay Bridge, where an accident lay ahead.

Oh, this is just great! Now I'm going to be late, I thought to myself.

Little did I know—that accident was no "accident." It put events in motion that would change my life forever . . .

The life of an agent in the United States Secret Service leaves little time for oneself. Structure and mission orientation are a way of life. An agent learns that early on when he or she accepts the invitation—and it *is* an invitation—after going through rigorous, comprehensive testing. From psychological workups and urine tests to the polygraph, everything is tested.

One of the rules all agents live by is if you're on time, you're late. Tardiness, when tolerated, is seen as a breakdown in preparedness. Agents learn that to be ultimately prepared, one makes it a point to use time to one's advantage. We prepared for everything, right down to the most advantageous time to eat (because sometimes we didn't get to).

Those of you reading this may be thinking, *That's crazy. How could anyone live in such a hyper-structured environment?* Well, it's easy when you report for duty each day with a mission that may require you to take or save a life. There's no room for error. Errors might cost lives. This is the way we trained; this is the way we lived. Being a member of the Secret Service involves sacrifice—it's a way of life that's not for everyone.

It also has its downside: There is little tolerance for anything or anyone who does not share the same value system. Inside the Service, life is golden; functioning outside can take its toll. The average agent is divorced at least once. Family life revolves around being on call 24/7/365.

The best part about being an agent? Your fellow agents always have your back . . . period.

I pulled into the parking garage at the World Trade Center, where our offices were located. I glanced down at my watch—8:43 a.m.

"Whew." I let out a sigh. *Less than fifteen minutes late. Not bad.*

I paged my supervisor (texting didn't exist yet) and let him know my status due to the accident. Today was a big day. We were preparing for the upcoming United Nations 50th Summit, and the New York Field Office was hosting the Police Meeting. (Prior to a big event, we typically met with the NYPD to coordinate the mission.) In 2001 the United States Secret Service had 2,300 agents worldwide, and we depended on the support and coordinated efforts of the local law enforcement agencies.

I quickly gathered my gear bag and walked inside the building, where I waited for the elevator. When the doors opened it was full of latecomers like me. I checked my watch—8:46 a.m. We silently acknowledged each other and then took the customary "strangers in an elevator" posture: everyone facing the door with their eyes upon the elevator floor reader located above the doors. The doors closed and the elevator started to move—and then unexpectedly the car shook and the lights flickered.

Oh great, now I'm getting stuck in the elevator, I thought.

There was a quizzical look in some of the other passengers' eyes. Then came the sound—as if a freight train was barreling down the tracks toward us. It grew louder and louder. The elevator car shot up like a missile and then abruptly stopped. It began bouncing up and down under the tension of the elevator's cable. Suddenly the doors flew open, and I was met with a hot blast of dust that blew me backward, literally taking my breath away.

As I regained my footing, I noticed the huge amount of debris that filled the mezzanine level of the WTC's North Tower, Tower One. Paper floated through the air, which was thick with dust from broken concrete. My automatic pilot kicked on. *A bomb,* I thought.

My specialized training as an agent afforded me the advantage of a "panic off, mission on" switch. At the United States Secret Service Training Center, our instructors would create scenarios where we constantly responded to emergency situations, drilling us over and over again. This created muscle memory in the brain. An emergency equaled calm, swift, decisive action. We had just been briefed on the World Trade Center bombing in 1993 in advance of the UN special event. In my mind a very calm voice said again, "Bomb."

Then the voice inside my head firmly said, "Get out."

I began to notice people doing the strangest things. One gentleman was trying to get back on the elevator, frantically pushing the down button. Others just stood there, completely paralyzed. I watched a security guard literally spin in circles. It was clear that it was every man (or woman) for himself (or herself).

In the elevator was a pregnant woman; she refused to leave the elevator. I looked her right in the eyes, identified myself as a United States Secret Service agent, and said, "Let's go—we're getting out."

I grabbed her hand, and we moved swiftly toward the escalator. She said nothing as we ran up the escalator. At the top of the escalator, we were now in 6 WTC, a place I had been every day since reporting for duty on October 20, 2000. As I paused for a moment, I noticed an emergency exit I had never used before. My instincts told me to go through it. It was a decision that would keep us shielded from the falling debris outside. 6 WTC was very unique in its construction. The building sat atop a narrower lobby level which created an overhang under which you could stand. It came in very handy on rainy days. On this day it would save lives.

Holding the hand of the pregnant woman, I looked at her and said, "This way."

Somewhere along the way we picked up a young black woman who was concerned because her daughter attended day care at the World Trade Center complex. "Follow me," I said.

Every day I passed that day care center on my way across the plaza from 6 WTC to my building, 7 WTC. As I pushed through the door with both women in tow, falling from the sky was a debris field of metal and rock and human body parts. As my brain adjusted to what I was seeing, it was as though we were on a movie set.

This isn't real. . . . Yes, it is, Sam. Keep moving.

I was in the middle of a war zone, but there was no identifiable enemy to shoot at. My gun stayed holstered. Then the young black woman saw the day care being evacuated. She ran to the door where the kids were being led out.

At this point we were completely shielded from the falling debris, and I walked purposefully with the pregnant lady toward the edge of 6 WTC. Ahead I could see the glass-covered walkway that connected the WTC Plaza to 7 WTC. It ran atop the busy street below. Upon reaching the edge of the building, I noticed that debris was falling everywhere, but it had not yet touched the walkway. I turned to the woman and said, "We're going over there."

She looked at me and uttered her first word: "Okay."

I could see my squad mates through the glass doors. They were motioning for me to come. I could see their lips moving, and I made out the word *run*. I paused for a moment amongst the rubble. I could see what looked like a wheel with metal connected to it. Rocks and dust and body parts continued to rain down. I looked up at the North Tower and clearly saw a man hanging out of the side of the building, waving his hands. Smoke was rushing out from behind him. I turned back and saw my squad mates. *Do I stay, or do I run?*

My squad mates continued to motion to me, mouthing the words, "Run! Run!" I could see my supervisor at the door. I saw her mouth form the words, "Come on, Sam," while waving her arm.

I turned to the pregnant lady. "Are you ready?" I asked.

She just stared at me. In her eyes I could see the uncertainty. The longer she stayed put, the harder it would be to get her to move. "We're going," I said.

I grabbed her hand and ran as hard and as fast as I could. My supervisor opened the door as she watched us run. I could now hear her and the other agents yelling, "Run! Come on, Sam, run!"

They pulled us inside.

We made it; we're safe, I thought.

Not quite . . .

My fellow agents and my supervisor asked if I was okay as they laid their hands on me as if making sure my limbs were all attached. I responded, "What the fuck is going on?"

Yes, it's true. In addition to sailors, cops are notorious for their foul mouths, and I was no exception. What made me nervous was my supervisor's response to my question.

"I don't know exactly. The news is reporting that a small plane crashed into the tower."

In my mind I was thinking, *Small plane, my ass*. The amount of debris and body parts I had seen indicated something much bigger.

At that point I started to cough. I felt like I had swallowed sand and there was nothing I could do to get it out. I pushed my way through the crowd to the small coffee shop located in the lobby of our building. This was a feat on its own—it was wall-to-wall humanity. Everyone was packed together, trying to get a glimpse of what was going on outside. I purchased some ice-cold juice, opened it, and guzzled half of it.

JUST ANOTHER DAY AT THE OFFICE

As I turned to make my way back to my squad mates, a second explosion rocked our building. I watched as the glass bowed to its breaking point. We were lucky because it held. As the glass moved so did the wall of people. I was pinned between the people in front of me and the countertop behind me. I could feel intense pressure against my spine. The wave of people kept pushing backward. The only thing I could think to do was yell, "Stop!"

I'd seen people severely injured and crushed to death on television in this same way, and I was not going to be one of them. I could barely take a breath. With everything I could muster, I yelled, "Stop! Stop moving!"

I immediately thought that bomb number two had just detonated. *We're next,* I told myself.

Building Seven was the third tallest building in the WTC complex, and it was full of agencies the public knew nothing about. I pushed my way through the crowd, intent on reaching the security guard who had a post inside the building. He was a very pleasant young man who greeted me daily with a big smile and a "Good morning, ma'am." Even though every time I would insist that he call me Sam, not "ma'am," the next day he would say "ma'am." There was something special about him. He made it a point to become everyone's friend. I often wonder what happened to him that day . . .

When I reached him I said, "I don't care what your orders are—we are evacuating this building now!"

Together with another agent, we started ushering people to the escalator and through the masked loading dock doors. The loading dock door was made to resemble the wall exactly, and it blended in so well you'd never know it was there. If you looked closely enough, you could see a small door handle, but most people walked by it day after day, never noticing.

There was an alternate exit ahead of us that led out onto the street. However, the debris from what we thought were explosions from a bomb continued to rain down, eliminating that as a possible evacuation route.

We walked through the corridor that led to our interrogation rooms. Hundreds of people squeezed through the narrow hallway. We finally came to a large, thick door marked Exit. Exiting the building onto the street brought a flood of smells, sounds, and sights that bombarded the senses. I could feel the adrenaline surging through my body. Debris was everywhere. We hurried past the Verizon Building and onto West Side Highway. Once people left the building, they started to scatter. Some walked around as if in a dream state, not knowing what to do.

Several agents and I stayed together as a group. We walked out onto the highway, hoping to get a better look at what was going on.

Out of nowhere a fellow agent's car came screeching to a halt behind us. We turned, startled by his skidding tires.

"Oh my God, are you guys okay? Did you see the planes?" he asked.

We looked at one another; we heard what he said, but no one responded. I finally broke the silence.

"What planes? Those were bombs."

"No, Sam. Planes flew into the towers," he replied.

I looked up, puzzled. "Planes?" I said.

I stared at the North Tower, trying to register what my eyes were seeing. As a trained investigator, the first rule of thumb before entering a crime scene was to look around and take in the whole scene. I began to see what looked like the shape of a plane—a big plane. As I studied it, the shape became clearer and clearer.

The agent broke the silence. "Oh my God! A plane just hit the Pentagon! We are being attacked!"

I looked back up at the North Tower. Smoke billowed from inside. In my head I repeated his words: *We are being attacked!*

My concentration was broken by a motorcade with full lights flashing and sirens blaring headed right toward the mayhem. I immediately recognized it as New York Mayor Rudy Giuliani's. The agent we were talking with told us he was leaving. He swung his car around and headed north, out of the city.

The group of agents and I managed to stay together. We crossed West Side Highway to get a better look at what was going on. We knew there were two explosions, but we couldn't see the South Tower, WTC Tower Two, from our vantage point. There were office buildings and high-rise residences across the street with views of the Hudson River. It was a nice spot where one could enjoy lunch outside in the shade and look out at the water.

As we walked, the ground proceeded to shake, and we heard a thundering noise overhead. We looked into each other's eyes and took off running toward the water. The sound grew louder and louder. In my mind I was prepared to jump into the Hudson if I needed to. With only the railing ahead, I looked up and saw two F-16 fighter jets. My heart pounded.

"What in God's name is going on?" I didn't realize I said this out loud.

THE SILENT FALL

An agent who was in my squad responded. "I don't know, but this is crazy."

We gathered ourselves and walked back toward West Side Highway to see more of what was happening. The South Tower came into view, and there was a huge gash in the right side of the building.

The second plane, I thought. We watched in silence as smoke and debris rained down from both WTC towers.

Suddenly our pagers began to go off one by one. The message read: "ALL NYFO AGENTS: If you are near Lower Manhattan, meet at the baseball field."

At first I thought it strange that someone was sending messages, and I wondered who it could be. But like good agents, we followed orders and proceeded to make our way three blocks north. The baseball field belonged to a school in Lower Manhattan; it was a little slice of pristine green heaven surrounded by tall buildings of steel and concrete. As we walked, we took in everything going on around us. The New York fire and police departments began arriving on the scene. People were everywhere. The towers continued to burn.

We entered the baseball field and made our way toward home plate. There were only a handful of us present. One of the supervisors was taking a mental accounting of who was there. From our position the North Tower was in full view, with the South Tower behind it. As we watched the North Tower burn, we saw what looked like a mannequin fall from high above. The agent standing next to me said, "Was that a . . . what *was* that?"

The human brain has the ability to play tricks on us. Based on previous pranks and hoaxes throughout the city, our brains were sending us the signal that we were seeing dummies or mannequins falling from the tower.

When I saw the second one, however, there was no mistaking what it was. We were so close we could feel the ground tremble when the bodies hit the concrete. After the tenth body, I stopped counting and tried to engage other agents in conversation. They were transfixed, not wanting to acknowledge what they were seeing. No one wanted to believe what we were witnessing. My supervisor said over and over again, "We're too close. This is too close."

We continued to watch the towers burn and people jump to their death. To this day I can only imagine the choice to jump or burn to death—it still makes me shudder.

I decided to call home, aware that my family needed to hear my voice. I dialed my mom, but the call wouldn't go through. I hit the redial button a few more times, but I got the same busy signal. I decided to try Steve, the man I had been dating for the last four months. I dialed his office number, and it connected. His front desk staff answered.

"White Oak Chiropractic, Christy speaking; how may I help you?"

"Christy, hey, it's Sam. Is Steve there?" I asked.

"Sam! Yes, hold on one second. I'll run to get Doc." Steve picked up the phone. "Sam, oh my God—are you okay? We've been watching on TV. Where are you?"

"I'm okay. I'm on a baseball field on West Side Highway."

Out of nowhere a police helicopter pilot decided to land exactly where we were standing. We scattered and ran to the fence line as it came closer to the ground. The noise of the helicopter made it impossible to hear anything Steve was saying. I yelled that

I would call him later and hung up, hoping he heard me.

As I walked along the fence line, trying to escape the dust the helicopter was kicking up, it happened. The South Tower was coming down. The roaring sound of bending, twisting metal, crumbling concrete, shattering glass, and screams filled the air. Then came the wall of dust. I took off running toward the school with the other agents.

As we stormed the front entrance, school administrators filed out of their offices, concerned at seeing armed agents entering their building. A few of the senior agents briefed them on what just occurred a few blocks away. The rest of us decided we needed to set up rescue and recovery efforts.

The male agents took off their dress shirts and undershirts and ripped them into pieces we could wrap around our mouths and noses. Despite our best efforts, there was no way to effectively keep from breathing in the asbestos and dust from the concrete, some of which was so fine it floated in the air. We were all prepared to leave when some of us realized that the people we were going to rescue needed to be brought to a central location.

Two other agents and I decided to stay behind to set up triage at the school. Technical first aid was part of the specialized training all Secret Service agents receive. We could patch a sucking chest wound if needed, so it made sense for us to set up an area where we could treat people until they could get to a hospital. The agents that ventured back down to the scene were prepared to bring people back to us. We immediately went into action and requested the help of all available school nurses along with their first-aid supplies. We decided that the gym would be our central holding place.

The school gym was perfect. It provided open space and there were mats we could use to keep people off the floor. We briefed the school principal, who was on board with our rescue efforts. He gave us access to all the school supplies and resources he had, including automatic external defibrillators. We were all set.

We waited to receive the victims. We waited and waited. No one was coming. *Surely there had to be victims,* I thought. We ventured outside into the dust-filled air, now mixed with thick black smoke. I could hear strange popping sounds. I could no longer see any of my fellow agents.

The principal of the school came running toward me. His superiors had contacted him and ordered an immediate evacuation of the school. Our rescue and triage efforts now became an evacuation effort. We hadn't realized that this school had a large special needs population—kids in wheelchairs, some with autism, and still others with disabilities both physical and mental.

The teachers started clearing the classrooms one by one as if conducting a fire drill—methodically but swiftly. This school had evacuation down. The two agents that were with me helped as we pushed wheelchairs and assisted those with physical challenges to move toward the exit that emptied out the back of the school, a block off of West Side Highway. We waited inside until the principal gave the all clear and confirmed that everyone was out. He thanked us for our help as he rushed to help the kids along.

Once outside the school, the two agents and I were now separated from the rest of the agents. As we walked toward West Side Highway, we noticed a young man who was quite large in stature. He was a student at the school, and several teachers were having trouble getting him to walk. They explained that the student was one of the special needs kids; he was frightened and didn't want to leave. We began slowly talking to the young man, pointing out that all of his friends were ahead of him. He stopped several times and refused to move.

We glanced back as we heard more unfamiliar sounds—popping, whistling, banging, and what could only be described as a very low growl that was getting louder and louder.

The agents and I made a "game time" decision. The only way we were going to get this young man out of danger was to carry him. He was well over six feet tall, too big to carry fireman-style. One of the agents grabbed the young man around the chest. I took a leg and the other agent grabbed the other one. We were off. One of the special needs aides approached us and said she worked with the young man in the classroom. I asked her to talk to him.

"Tell him we're helping him. Tell him we're friends and he's safe."

The low growl we had been hearing suddenly became very loud. We all turned to see the North Tower begin to implode.

"Go! Go! Go!" I yelled.

We moved as fast as we could as we watched the cloud of dust grow closer to us, heading straight up West Side Highway.

"Don't look back, just go!" I yelled.

Everything was so incredibly loud around us. We went as fast as our bodies would take us. The stress and strain of carrying this very large young man made every muscle burn as they filled with lactic acid. Once beyond the enormous dust cloud, we stopped. We turned around and immediately noticed the hole in one of the most famous skylines in the world. Both the North and South Towers were gone. In their place was thick black smoke and twisted metal. A firefighter came into view. He was covered in dust. A small stream of blood ran down his forehead from underneath his helmet.

JUST ANOTHER DAY AT THE OFFICE

Oh my God, I thought, *where are my fellow agents who went to pull people out?*

The two agents and I looked at each other. Without saying a word, we resumed carrying our young friend. The firefighters saw us struggling and came over to help. I asked the one who was bleeding if he was okay, and without hesitating he grabbed part of the leg I was holding. We kept walking. I noticed a cameraman taking pictures. Couldn't he see that we needed help?

Little did I know, one of those pictures would appear in *People* magazine and immortalize us forever.

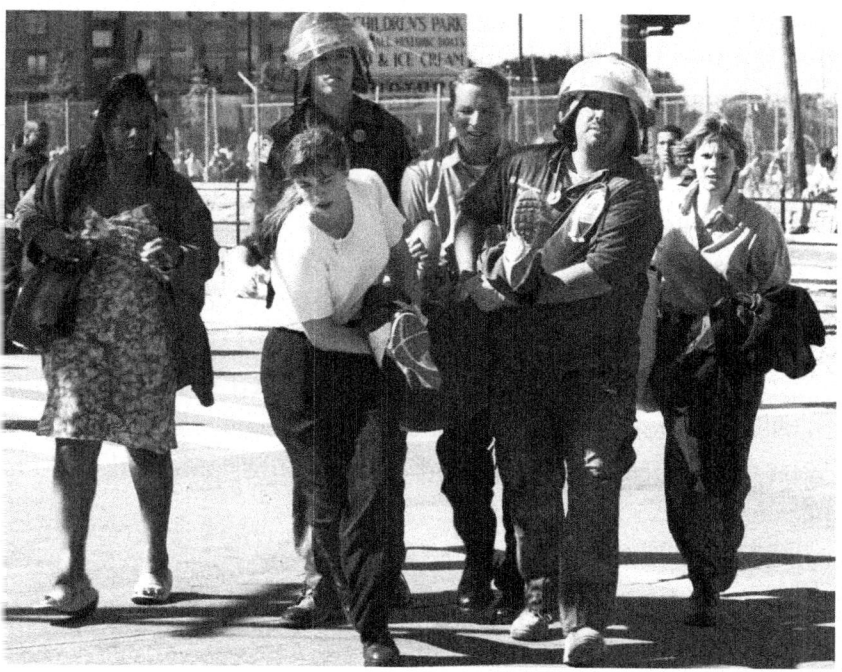

Myself (far right) along with my two agent partners and two firefighters, as we carry the young man we evacuated from the school after 1 WTC collapsed. His aide is on the far left. (Photograph courtesy Alecsey Boldeskul)

25

An ambulance came screaming toward us. It turned around so its back doors were facing us. Paramedics rushed over to us with a stretcher. We loaded the young man on the stretcher, and the bleeding firefighter took a seat on the edge of the bumper. One of the paramedics handed him a bottle of water; he removed his helmet and poured the water over his head.

We instructed the young man's aide to go to the hospital with him. She quickly jumped into the back of the ambulance and held his hand.

After making sure the three of us were okay, the paramedics jumped into the ambulance and drove away. There we stood in the middle of West Side Highway, looking at the burning wreckage and smoke. A steady stream of people filed passed us in a daze, some completely covered in thick white dust.

Our pagers beeped again. "How the heck?" I said. "Who could be sending out messages?"

The screen read, "ALL NYFO AGENTS: If you are on the west side of the city, meet at West 63rd Street Pier."

We looked around to see where we were. We were between West 21st and 22nd Streets. We had walked with that young man in tow for almost two miles. As we began heading toward West 63rd Street, the lactic acid started to dissipate and walking became easier.

TWO

HEADING HOME

THE TWO AGENTS and I arrived at the West 63rd Street Pier and went inside. I was relieved to see several supervisors and most of the agents we had thought were still down at what would come to be known as "Ground Zero." We were told to go upstairs to the bathrooms and get cleaned up and then grab something to drink—the Pier 63 staff had arranged sodas and water for us.

I remember how good the air conditioning felt as I walked upstairs and entered the bathroom. "Oh my gosh!" I said, startled at my appearance. I was covered in dust: There was dust in my hair, on my clothes, on my face. I ran my fingers back and forth through my hair until the dust stopped falling. I wiped my clothes off, then washed my face. The cool water felt so good as it splashed on my face!

I walked back out into the main room where most of the other agents were. I grabbed a soda and sat in the corner against the windows. Most of us sat in silence while the supervisors began to take attendance and try to figure out who was unaccounted for. A young agent who had not been in the field office very long arrived, completely covered in dust. Her hair and skin were the color of concrete. I overheard her saying that she had to break a storefront window and jump through it to escape the wall of dust and debris.

"Okay, listen up," a supervisor said. "We've arranged for the Park Police to take you guys that live in New Jersey over to Hoboken where you'll meet up with agents from the New Jersey Field Office. They are driving all the available cars and will get each of you home. Everyone go down to the dock and wait for instructions on boarding the boats."

With a sigh of relief, I grabbed my stuff and filed out of Pier 63 onto the dock with several of my squad mates. Our supervisor came over and asked if we had seen certain agents who had not checked in anywhere, but all we could account for was ourselves. We wondered if they were okay . . .

On the pier we couldn't help but stare at where the towers once stood. Thick black smoke was all that was visible. Out of nowhere there was a loud grumbling sound that took us by surprise. We couldn't determine where it was coming from. It grew louder and louder. We all hit the deck as if something was going to come tumbling down on our heads. We looked up and saw two F-16 fighter jets roaring by. They were flying so low we could see the markings on the planes. All at once we let out a cheer. "Yeah! Go get em, U-S-A!"

The entire island of New York City was surrounded by military fighter jets. They circled Manhattan continuously for hours, flying in formation, two at a time.

The Park Police arrived with the first boat to ferry us across to Hoboken, New Jersey. I piled in with some of my squad mates. All eyes were fixed on the raging fires and black smoke that trailed off over the Hudson River toward New Jersey. I was trying to comprehend what occurred, but it seemed like a dream. I tried to tell myself that tomorrow I'd wake up and everything would

HEADING HOME

be fine. Logically I knew it would not. Tomorrow would never be the same—and neither would I.

As we pulled away from the pier, we donned life jackets and stood silently watching the new skyline that had formed in front of us. When we reached Hoboken, we were met by agents from the New Jersey Field Office. We figured out where everyone lived and broke up into small groups. Five of us piled into a sedan headed south on the New Jersey Turnpike for Metuchen, Edison, and New Brunswick. I sat on the lap of one of my squad mates. Not ideal, but I was going home.

We didn't get far before the New Jersey State Police decided to close the Turnpike. Although we were in a vehicle loaded with law enforcement officers, they refused to allow us to proceed. Plan B: side roads. Route 1 was the only other option that made sense, so our driver swung the car around, and we were once again on our way. The streets were empty, with an occasional car driving by in the opposite direction. I looked at the clock in the car—4:33 p.m. It was the first time I had checked the time since arriving to work at 8:43 a.m.

The agent from the New Jersey Field Office started asking questions about the attack. We gave very short and direct answers. At one point the car was silent except for the few directions the agent needed in order to drop us off one by one.

"Oh shit," I cursed. "The keys to my apartment and my POV were in my G-Ride."

We referred to our personal vehicles as POVs: Privately Owned Vehicles. Our G-Rides, or government cars, were used each day in conjunction with our duties. Although we were federal agents technically on duty 24/7/365, we had very strict rules as to who could travel in our G-Rides and when we could use them. If we were not on a protective assignment, in the midst of conducting an investigation, or on another job-related function, we were prohibited from using our G-Rides.

My G-Ride was part of the rubble heap under the North Tower.

"Come to my house, Sam. Call your landlord, and my wife and I will drive you home," replied one of my squad mates. We lived ten minutes from each other in Edison, New Jersey, and often gave each other rides to the office.

"Thanks—I really appreciate it," I replied.

We pulled up in front of my squad mate's house and said our good-byes to our fellow agents. My squad mate and I entered his house, and he and his wife embraced. I felt like the proverbial fifth wheel.

I went into the other room and called my landlord.

"Oh my God, Sam! I'm so glad to hear your voice! Are you okay? What do you need?" I had the best landlord in the world. He rented a beautiful 800-plus-square-foot fully carpeted one-bedroom second floor walk-up to me for practically nothing. At twenty-nine years old, I was banking money each month.

"I need a new set of keys to the apartment," I said.

"No problem—I'm on my way. I'll meet you in twenty minutes," he replied.

I walked into the other room where my squad mate and his wife were talking. "My landlord said he'll be at my place in twenty minutes."

"No problem. Let me grab my keys and we'll go," said my squad mate.

On the drive to my apartment, we said very little to each other; we were still trying to comprehend what had occurred. We pulled into my apartment complex and up to the front door of my building. My landlord was already waiting for me. I thanked my squad mate, closed the door to his truck, and waved good-bye.

My landlord gave me a big hug. "I'm so glad you're okay, Sam. I knew you worked right there, and I was so worried," he said.

"Thanks. It's good to be home," I replied.

I looked at my watch. It was 5:00 p.m. The time had flown by. I followed behind my landlord as he opened the first set of doors with the new key. We walked up the stairs to my apartment, and he put the second key in the door. It opened easily. He handed me the keys.

"Thanks so much. You're a Godsend," I said.

"Sam, I think you're the Godsend," he said. "I can only imagine what it was like, but I know you, and I know you helped a lot of people today. You're like a hero."

"I was just doing my job, but thanks," I replied. I was very uncomfortable with the word *hero*. There were so many more lives that could have been saved. *What kind of hero feels helpless?* I thought.

My landlord asked if I needed anything else. He even offered me dinner, which I declined with a smile. "You're a hero" kept playing over and over in my head.

I walked him to the door, went to the window, and watched him leave. *Ah, quiet,* I thought as I sat in my kitchen. It dawned on me a few minutes later that I had to get replacement keys to my POV. I picked up the phone and dialed 411. (This was before cell phones could search the Internet; it was either the White Pages or Information.) I got the number for the closest Honda dealership, which was just up the road and thankfully open for one more hour.

I explained to the service manager what happened, and he told me come right over with the title to my car and he would cut me a new key.

I went downstairs to my neighbor's apartment. We had been neighbors for almost a year, but because of my crazy travel schedule, we basically passed each other in the hallway and that was that. I was either coming or going.

"Hey there. I'm your neighbor upstairs. My name's Sam," I said.

"Of course. Hi. What's up?" she replied.

"I was wondering if you could take me up to the Honda dealership. I don't know if you know what I do. I'm a Secret Service agent." I showed her my credentials, which I somehow had managed to hold onto. "I lost my car keys when Tower One collapsed on my government car. I just got home, and the manager at the dealership said he could cut me a new key if I came up now."

She stared back at me as if she hadn't comprehended what I had said.

"Wait . . . Sam—you were there today?" she asked.

"Yes. I was in Tower One when the plane hit. I was on my way to work."

"Holy shit, girl!" she yelled.

I smiled back. I hadn't heard anyone say that since college.

"Hang on, I'll get my keys," she said.

We got into her car and drove down the road to the dealership.

"What do you do?" I asked.

"I'm a teacher. The schools let out early today with everything going on," she replied.

"What grade are you in?" I asked. (My aunt was a teacher, and she always said that when you meet a teacher, you ask what grade they're *in* instead of what grade they *teach*.)

"Fifth," she responded.

I went on automatic pilot again. Even though I answered a bunch of her questions, it was as if I had gone somewhere else while still remaining present enough to comprehend and respond.

We arrived at the Honda dealership. I walked into the service area, met the manager, presented the title to my car, and he returned a few minutes later with a new key.

"Thank you very much. I appreciate your help," I said as I turned toward the door.

"No problem, ma'am," he responded.

I was just about to walk out when I heard him say, "Excuse me—ma'am?"

I turned to see the manager's hand extended. "Thank you, ma'am, for your service. I'm glad you made it out," he said.

I shook his hand, turned around, and walked out the door. My neighbor was waiting patiently for me in her car. We left the dealership and headed back to the apartment complex. On the way my neighbor continued to ask me questions. I responded consciously, but mentally I was somewhere else. I knew she was talking, but I do not remember hearing a word.

We pulled into the parking lot and got out of the car. I thanked her again for helping me out.

"Are you kidding me? This was no problem at all. If you need anything, you just ask. You're a hero," she said.

There was that word again. "Thank you, but I was just doing my job," I responded.

We walked into our building. I went upstairs to my apartment and let myself in.

I put the keys on the counter and sat down in my kitchen. I was happy to be in a safe, quiet place. I noticed that my ears were ringing—the kind of ringing you experience after you've gone to a really loud rock concert. I picked up my landline and dialed Steve's number. The phone line cut off. I hung up and pressed redial. The same thing happened. "Come on, phone, please connect," I said. The third time I dialed, it finally connected. Steve answered quickly. "Hi, Sam. Where are you?"

"I'm finally back at my apartment," I replied.

"Are you okay?" Steve asked.

"I think so. I'm just sitting in my kitchen. The phone lines are all screwed up," I answered.

"Sam, do you want me to come up?" he asked.

"Tonight?" I asked in return.

"Yes. I'll leave as soon as I get a bag packed."

"Are you sure?" It was a fairly long drive from Maryland.

"I'm very sure. You shouldn't be by yourself," he said with concern in his voice. It was if he could tell that I was somehow acting differently. I accepted his offer gratefully. I looked forward to having him hold me in his arms. I hung up the phone and felt a sense of relief wash over me. I took a deep breath and resumed sitting quietly.

My serenity was broken by the ringing of my kitchen telephone. It startled me. "Hello?"

"Sam! I'm so glad I got through! It's so good to hear your voice. I thought you were gone. I just watched your building come down," the voice on the other end of the line said.

"Hey, Scott. It's great to hear your voice, too."

Scott was my best friend. He and I met in junior high school. We saw each other almost every day from that moment on. We remained close through college and law school. He had moved to Boston, but we stayed in touch. Although the Secret Service had me traveling nonstop, we managed to stay in touch via email and the occasional phone call.

"The phone lines are a mess. I've been trying you for a while. When I saw your building collapse, I panicked," he said.

"You mean Towers One and Two—my building didn't get hit," I responded.

"You worked in Building Seven, right?" he asked.

When I said yes, he went on. "Your building just came down. I'm watching it on TV."

I went over to the television and turned it on. I hadn't realized that when the North Tower collapsed, it sheared off the front of Building Seven. I watched as the news replayed Building Seven's collapse.

"Oh no," I said as I sat down on the couch.

I went on to tell Scott what I'd been through. He was silent as I recounted the day's events.

"Oh my God, Sam. I'm so glad you're okay."

After I hung up I decided that I'd better start calling home to check in with my family. I had been able to reach my mom before the Towers came down, but not after; I knew she would be concerned. Her line was busy. I tried again. "All circuits are busy now," said the recorded voice on the other end.

I kept hitting the redial button until I was able to get through.

"Hi, Mom. I'm back at my apartment," I said as soon as she answered.

"Oh, honey, I'm so glad to hear your voice. I was so worried. I didn't know what happened to you when the Towers fell," she said.

"Yeah, it was pretty crazy, Mom." I filled her in on the details.

Prior to the Towers coming down, my mom had acted as a liaison. Part of the preparation for the UN's 50th anniversary event was having armored vehicles brought up from Washington, DC. They were stored in the underground parking under Tower One behind locked gates. The security for the vehicles was provided by several agents from the Special Services division. When they received the text pages after we evacuated, they met us at the ball field. My cell phone was one of just a few that was able to connect. I telephoned my mom at her office to let her know I had made it out of my building, and I asked if she would take the names and numbers of the agents' family members and call them so they'd know their loved ones were safe. I passed the phone to the first agent, who relayed his information. Then, one by one, they passed the phone until all of them had given their information to my mom.

"Thanks for helping this morning, Mom. The guys really appreciated it."

"It was my pleasure, sweetie," she responded. "Did you get a chance to talk to Steve?" she asked.

"Yes. He's coming up tonight," I responded.

"Oh . . . well, he certainly cares for you," she said. I could sense that, while she was relieved I wasn't going to be by myself, she didn't totally approve of Steve staying overnight. I don't like to call my mom old-fashioned, but she is not a fan of two unwed people spending the night together. Even at twenty-nine, with my own apartment and living independently in another state, she did not approve.

"Mom, come on, I'm almost thirty years old. Are we going to keep this going? Steve and I have spent many a night together—you know that."

"I know, honey. I just worry, that's all. All I can say is after what you went through today, he's either going to run or marry you," she said with a touch of laughter in her voice.

We said our good-byes and hung up. I took my suit jacket off and went into the bathroom. As soon as I closed the door, I felt strangely uncomfortable. I opened the door and the uncomfortable feeling went away. *That's weird*, I thought. I turned on the shower, kicked off my shoes, closed the door to the bathroom—and the strange feeling returned. This time it was stronger. My heart began to race. I quickly opened the door again. My heart rate returned to normal, and I could breathe more easily.

I turned the water off in the shower and returned to the kitchen. *This is so bizarre. Why can't I close the door?* I shook my head and poured myself a glass of water. I'd barely eaten or had anything to drink all day, yet I wasn't hungry or even thirsty.

The phone rang again. It was my uncle. Uncle Lee always brought a smile to my face, and I enjoyed our conversations. As a child I remember he was always at our house, ready to play.

Back in the '70s he was the human jungle gym. My sister and I would hang from both of his arms. At 6'3" tall, with biceps that rivaled the World's Strongest Man competitors, my uncle was the biggest and boldest person I knew. He could throw a tennis ball so high in the air that it would disappear against the backdrop of the sky. He got his chiseled physique from chiseling marble—literally. After his brief military service, he became a conservator at Washington, DC's famous Hershorn Museum and became a sculptor himself. Some of his pieces weighed over 400 pounds and required a small crane to move them. He had been there for every milestone in my life.

"Hey there, kiddo. It's good to hear your voice. What a mess, huh?" he said.

"Things are so crazy," I responded.

"I spoke with your mom earlier, and she filled me in on some of the details. I'm watching the coverage on TV. There was another plane that crashed in Pennsylvania. They're reporting that its intended target was most likely the White House."

"Holy crap. This was obviously an attack on us," I responded.

"Yes, I can only imagine how this is going to play out." He asked me if I was watching TV, and I told him no, that I was just trying to process it all.

Are you okay?" he asked.

"Yeah, I'm okay," I said. I did not tell him about being unable to close the bathroom door.

"Okay, I'll let you go. Anything I can do?" he said.

"Yes—do you mind calling around and letting everyone know I'm in my apartment and I'm fine? I need a break from the phone."

"Sure thing," he said, and we hung up.

HEADING HOME

I resumed sitting in the kitchen. It seemed like a long time had passed when the phone rang again. I looked up and the clock showed that only ten minutes had gone by. It was Steve. He said it had taken several tries to finally get through. "The closer I get, the worse the signal," he reported.

Steve was almost at the Delaware Memorial Bridge. He was very proud of the time he was making, since there was practically no one else on the road.

"What time do you think you'll arrive?" I asked.

"Certainly by nine, barring any issues. I'm driving eighty-five miles an hour!"

"Eighty-five!" I said, impressed. Traveling I-95 North over the years had become increasingly worse due to the traffic. Any trips to and from New Jersey were usually at five in the morning or nine at night. I couldn't remember the last time a trip at 7:40 p.m. on a weeknight had not been met with multiple curse words because traffic was at a standstill.

"I wo-do-ta-na—" Steve's cell signal was cutting out. I was only able to capture every other word before the line went silent. A few minutes later he called back to say he was already at Exit Three and explained that there were signs everywhere saying Exit Ten (my exit) was the last exit before the New Jersey Turnpike was closed to traffic.

Steve was born in Brooklyn and at age seven moved to Bergen County, New Jersey, just across the George Washington Bridge. There was always plenty of traffic on the New Jersey Turnpike; it was never closed, and it was extremely rare to be able to drive eighty-five miles an hour.

On many a trip back and forth to Maryland, I had been

stopped by New Jersey state troopers. As a federal agent I traveled with my gun on me, my credentials always on my dashboard. We were taught to always have our credentials on the dash because it eliminated having to take our hands off the steering wheel.

After a trooper introduced himself, I'd politely reply, "Federal agent traveling armed. My credentials are on the dash. I'm going to reach for them with my right hand and give them to you." The trooper would take my credentials, look at them, and normally respond by thanking me and wishing me a good day or evening. There was a mutual respect between law enforcement agencies—a bond that grew stronger after 9/11 and continues to run deep.

Steve arrived just before nine o'clock, and I buzzed him in. I opened my apartment door and fell into his arms. I had missed his hugs. At only 5'8" inches tall, years of powerlifting gave him broad, strong shoulders. We hugged for what seemed like a long time, and he kissed me gently. We had no idea at the time, but his visit solidified our future relationship together.

I took his hand, and we went into the kitchen. "Hey, I have to ask you a question, because the weirdest thing is happening," I said.

"Anything," he responded.

I hesitated. "Um, I need to take a shower, but I can't close the door to the bathroom. I don't know why. Would you sit in the bathroom with me?" I asked.

Steve looked puzzled. I imagined he thought, *A United States Secret Service Agent who can't take a shower?*

"I know it sounds weird, but I just get a really uncomfortable feeling," I said, trying to explain.

With Steve in the bathroom with me, I got into the shower,

pulled the curtain closed, and let the warm water run over my face. It felt so good. But suddenly I could feel my heart start to race. I opened my eyes. "Steve, are you there?"

"Yes, I'm right here, Sam."

I pulled the curtain back and saw him sitting on the floor in the doorway. Every time I closed my eyes, the uncomfortable feeling in my chest returned. I felt relieved when I finished. I turned off the water, Steve handed me a towel, and I changed into my bedclothes.

For the first time since breakfast, I started to think about food.

"You've eaten, right, Sam?"

"No, I haven't been hungry till now." It was definitely not like me to go without eating an entire day. My workouts usually had me eating every three to four hours. I went into the kitchen and opened the fridge. I found half of a leftover chicken breast. I looked in the cabinets and saw a small amount of angel hair pasta. *Perfect*, I thought. I put a pot of water on the stove to boil. Steve began to ask me questions about what happened. Just like with my neighbor, I heard him talking and responded, but I had gone somewhere else in my mind.

"Sam, the water is boiling." Steve broke my mind's silence.

"Huh? Oh, thanks."

"Sam, are you sure you're okay?" Steve asked.

"I guess I just must be tired or something . . . I don't know," I said as I put the pasta into the boiling water.

The phone rang. "It's your mom," Steve said, looking at the caller ID. "Hi, Vicki. I arrived about an hour ago, and Sam is making herself some dinner." He told my mom how strange it was to be one of the few cars on the road, with all access to New

York City closed off. As I listened I could only imagine what was happening in Washington, DC.

I talked to my mom briefly and told her I was making dinner.

"It's after ten o'clock. You're just eating dinner?" she said with concern in her voice. I assured her I would eat and stay in touch. She asked me to pass the phone back to Steve.

"Steve, take care of my baby," I heard her say.

Next my grandparents called to check up on me. I asked them how things were in DC. I started shoveling food into my mouth as they explained that the government told everyone except essential personnel to go home and stay there unless it was absolutely necessary to go out. I hadn't seen any footage of the crash at the Pentagon, and my grandparents explained how the plane took out one entire side of the building. The officials were still trying to determine how many people died.

My grandfather, Papa Harry, was a decorated World War II veteran. He was in the Battle of Guadalcanal. He had been on two Navy transport ships, both of which were blown up when the Japanese purposely crashed their planes into them. He had spent days in the water. I could only imagine what he had gone through. I knew he understood what I had just experienced. I knew it had to bring back memories for him. I don't think he ever thought he would see planes used this way again.

"How are you, Papa Harry?" I asked.

"I'm fine, sweetheart. I want you to take care of yourself," he replied.

My grandfather never spoke of the war again after 9/11. He took his memories to the grave with him five days after Steve and I were married.

I hung up the handset and stood quietly staring out the window. I put the last bite of food in my mouth and walked over to the sink to rinse the plate and put it in the dishwasher.

"What do you want to do, Sam?" Steve asked. My pager interrupted my answer. "All NYFO Agents: Mandatory meeting Thursday 9/13, 1000hrs, JFK Airport Services Building 3."

I read Steve the message. "Do you want me to drive you?" he asked.

"I don't know. Let me make a call," I responded.

I called one of my squad mates to see if he could shed some light on it. Since he was a senior agent, I told him that Steve was here and asked if he thought it would be a problem if Steve drove me to the meeting. He didn't seem to think it would be a problem. "Worst case, Sam, he drops you off and picks you up when we're through," he said.

Suddenly I felt tired. I took Steve's hand and led him to the bedroom. I was relieved to get at least one day's rest without having to worry about being somewhere. We climbed into bed. I rested my head on Steve's chest with my arm wrapped around him.

Sometime during the middle of the night, I screamed out. "No! No!"

Steve woke me up. "Sam, Sam, it's a dream. Wake up."

I was covered in sweat. "What in the heck?"

"What were you dreaming?" Steve asked.

"I don't know," I said, trying to catch my breath.

He wrapped his strong arms around me, and I put my head on his chest. At some point I drifted back to sleep.

THREE

THE NEW NORMAL

THE NEXT MORNING I awoke to the sound of the trash truck banging the dumpster around. I felt as if I were drugged. I rolled over in bed; I barely had any energy. *Coffee*, I thought. I had set the timer the night before, so there was a full pot waiting for me. I turned to Steve.

"Good morning," he said.

"Hmm," I muttered back. I was not a morning person, and Steve knew not to say anything until I had downed at least one cup of coffee. I dragged myself into the kitchen and poured myself a huge mug. I stayed in the kitchen, staring out the window and deliberately taking large sips. My philosophy was to get caffeinated as quickly as possible because you never know what's coming next. Steve came up behind me and put his arms around my waist.

"You had some kind of dream last night," he said.

"I know—I'm sorry I woke you," I responded, pouring mug number two.

"Do you remember anything?"

I told him I didn't remember a thing. I switched the subject to breakfast. My omelets and oatmeal were legendary with my family and friends, and I happily prepared some now for Steve, who was eager to turn on the television.

"If you don't mind, could you keep the volume down? I don't think the news can report any better than my firsthand experience yesterday."

I took a deep breath and sighed, happy to wake up and have my mind on making a delicious breakfast. The thought of my building coming down did intrigue me, however. I asked Steve to let me know when they showed Building Seven coming down.

The water for the oatmeal began to boil. I poured the oatmeal in, turned the heat down to a simmer, and placed the lid on top of the pot with just enough room for the steam to escape. I had watched my Grandma Nan and my mom cook this way so the pot wouldn't boil over.

"Hey Sam, it's coming up next," Steve said.

I made sure the heat was turned down and the top of the lid was open enough so when I stepped away I would not come back to a mess on the stovetop. I walked into the living room and sat down next to Steve. He took my hand.

The news showed each WTC Tower collapse into one another. First the South Tower, then the North, then Building Seven.

"Son of a bitch. He fucking did it!" I blurted out angrily.

"Who did what?" Steve said as I stared at the television. When I didn't answer, he asked again. "Sam, who did what?"

I turned to Steve. "What?"

"You said, 'He fucking did it.' Who did what?"

"Have you ever heard of Khalid Sheikh Mohammed?" I said.

"No. Who is he?" Steve asked.

Khalid Sheikh Mohammed was the Islamic terrorist responsible for the World Trade Center bombings in 1993. He detonated a huge truck bomb under the North Tower. His objective was to blow up the North Tower and have it crash into the South Tower. Six people died and a thousand were injured.

Steve looked at me with his mouth wide open. "Wait a second," Steve said. "They didn't catch him?"

"Nope," I said.

The federal law enforcement community knew that several others helped the sheikh pull off the bombing in 1993. Several agencies and our military had been after them for a while.

"He obviously succeeded with his original plan."

"Damn it!" I yelled.

I smelled the oatmeal and ran into the kitchen just in time to take the oatmeal off the flame. I took out a wooden spoon and stirred. *Ah, now that's perfection.*

I put a dollop of sweet crème butter on top and put the lid back on to let it cool. There is nothing worse than burning the roof of your mouth on scalding hot oatmeal. I grabbed the eggs from the fridge, cracked them into a bowl and whisked away until a lovely froth formed on top. I put some butter in the skillet and poured the golden froth into the skillet.

"Here you go," I said as I placed the eggs and oatmeal down on the coffee table in front of Steve.

"Smells delicious."

"Enjoy," I responded, returning to the kitchen to grab another cup of coffee and a bagel I had started for myself.

Bing—the toaster announced that my bagel was done. I took my favorite cream cheese from the fridge, grabbed a knife, and coated the perfectly toasted bagel with a delicate layer. I put one half of the bagel on top of the other and took a bite. I never ate my bagel one half at a time. When both halves were put together,

THE SILENT FALL

I could eat faster. It seemed as if everything about my life was geared toward getting things done as efficiently and quickly as possible.

I joined Steve on the couch, and we watched in silence as the news replayed the sequence of the attacks. There was footage from each plane being driven first into the Towers and then into the Pentagon, followed by the Towers collapsing, and finally Building Seven coming down. The news then went live to what was now being called "Ground Zero." The news reported that a crash site had been found in Shanksville, Pennsylvania, and there was speculation that it was the missing United Airlines Flight 93 which had been headed to Washington, DC.

I finished my bagel while Steve was still eating. "Want anything else from the kitchen?" I asked as I got up from the couch.

"More orange juice, please," Steve responded. I refilled his glass and grabbed a fresh mug of coffee before returning to the living room.

"So let me get this straight," Steve said. "This terrorist guy did the bombing in 1993?"

"Yes," I responded.

"And how do we know this?"

"From intel that was put together from the crime scene. We were just re-briefed on it yesterday."

"What intel?"

"I can't tell you that," I responded. "But we are 100 percent sure that Khalid Sheikh Mohammed was responsible for the '93 bombing, and it looks like he is responsible for this, too."

"How do you know that?" Steve asked.

"Like I said before. His main objective was to collapse the

Towers back in 1993. Do you think what happened yesterday is a coincidence? They took their time in planning this one."

"They?"

"Yes, they. Khalid Sheikh Mohammed was the ring leader, and the others carried it out."

Steve just sat there looking at me. I could see his brain going a mile a minute.

Our conversation was interrupted by my pager sounding from the bedroom where I'd left it the night before. I scurried to the bedroom and read, "ALL NYFO AGENTS REPORT TO YOUR SQUAD LEADERS."

I picked up the phone and dialed my squad leader's number. She answered on the fourth ring.

"CJ here," she said.

"Hey, it's Sam. Just got the page."

"Hey, Sam. Thanks for calling in. How are you doing?"

"Umm, I guess okay."

She gave clear instructions to check in with her daily, and she wanted to make sure I had spoken with my family. Then she asked me the strangest question.

"Listen," she said "have you seen or heard from Mark or Ann?"

Mark and Ann were the two newest members of our squad. They also happened to be the youngest, so naturally there was concern.

"I was with Ann yesterday until we got to Hoboken. Never saw Mark."

"Hmm . . . we keep calling their land lines and cell phones, but we can't reach them. And you were with Ann yesterday?"

"Yes. We took the police boat to Hoboken, and then she got

into one of the New Jersey agents' car with some others. Mark lives close by, but I don't remember seeing him on the boat with us."

"Okay. If you hear from either of them, will you please tell them to call me ASAP?"

"You bet. No problem," I responded.

"Thanks, Sam. See you tomorrow morning."

I hung up the phone and went back into the living room where Steve was still fixated on the TV. I explained that we were missing one agent from my squad and another was not answering her pager or phone.

Steve had a look of concern on his face. "Come here," he said, patting the empty space on the couch next to him. He put his arm around me and drew me closer to him. I put my head on his shoulder and closed my eyes. We sat quietly for what seemed like an eternity. I felt safe and secure.

The news broke the quiet of the moment. I picked my head up off of Steve's shoulder as the news anchor spoke. "Here are new images coming to us. We must warn you, these images are graphic in nature." They showed images of the South Tower burning and people jumping. It was as if a switch had been flipped inside me. My heart began to race, and I began to sweat. "Oh God," I said, as I closed my eyes and buried my head in Steve's chest.

"Oh God. Sam, I'm so sorry. Shit, where's the remote?" he said as he searched the cushions of the couch. He turned off the TV as fast as he could. He held me close. My head was buried in his chest. I felt my heartbeat start to slow down. I took a deep breath and let it out.

Steve took my face in his hands. "Sam, are you okay?" he asked.

"Yeah . . . that was weird," I replied.

Steve pulled me in close again and wrapped his arms around me. I melted into him. My gaze drifted to the window, and I stared at the trees as they swayed in the breeze. Then, out of the blue, I felt the need to move. "Let's go for a walk," I said.

We both threw on some workout clothes. I put my gun into my fanny pack and clipped my pager onto the strap.

"You need your gun to take a walk?" Steve asked.

"Of course. After yesterday you can never be too prepared."

Steve stood there for a second with a confused look on his face. I had never taken my gun with me to work out. Walk, run, or whatever—it was usually the only time I happily shed the weight of my Sig Sauer P229 .357.

We walked out the front door into the sunshine and the crisp September air. It was unusually quiet for this time of the morning. Typically there were always cars and school buses hustling up and down the road. I also noticed that the sky was quiet. Living only three exits from Newark International Airport, there was a continuous stream of planes overhead either preparing to land or taking off. The stillness was peaceful and calming.

Steve and I held hands as we walked to a nearby school. It was closed. We passed a few storefronts. Everyone had the television on. After my experience earlier, I knew that watching the specific coverage of what happened yesterday on the television was not going to be part of my daily routine for a while.

We got back to my apartment. We couldn't believe that most of the day had already passed. It was nearly four o'clock. I suggested an early dinner. "Why don't you pick the place, and I'll go shower," I said.

I went into the bathroom and turned on the shower to start the hot water. I was grabbing my robe from the bedroom when suddenly I heard a very low grumbling sound that seemed to grow louder by the second until it was overhead. My heart raced, and I crouched down almost under my bed. "What the hell is that?" I screamed.

Steve came running and found me on the floor. He bent down and covered me with his body.

"It's okay, Sam, it's two F-16s," he said as he hugged me.

"Damn it. Okay. I'm okay," I said angrily.

"Here, let me help you," Steve said.

"I don't need help!" I barked back at Steve.

The word *help* did not register. *Why am I in need of help?* I thought. *I'm not injured. I'm not bleeding. I'm not . . . why am I on the floor?*

Steve stood there looking at me.

"I'm sorry. I didn't mean that." I got up and hugged Steve. "Thank you."

I broke our embrace and went into the bathroom again. I looked at myself in the mirror and shook my head as if to say, "No way, girl. Get yourself together."

I closed the bathroom door and immediately opened it again. *Music*, I thought. I asked Steve to turn on my favorite radio station. We were both big classic rock fans—almost anything in the genre suited us, from Yes and Foreigner to the Doobie Brothers. We enjoyed it all and went to many concerts together when I was able to come back to Maryland.

We enjoyed concerts at Wolf Trap the most. During the summer months all the big headliners would come to Wolf Trap.

You could sit inside the amphitheater or out on the lawn. Any seat was the "best seat in the house." One evening we saw Foreigner; they put on an amazing show. Steve had a friend who worked backstage, and we got to meet the band. They signed the only thing I had available, my Secret Service water bottle.

Stevie Ray Vaughn was playing on the radio, and Steve cranked up the volume. I jumped in the shower and danced my way clean. The music definitely helped, and even though I still couldn't close the bathroom door, it helped me to not focus on being in an enclosed space.

I got out of the shower and dried off. "Your turn," I said to Steve.

Steve walked over and kissed me before disappearing behind the bathroom door. I smiled and grooved my way into the bedroom to dress. It was the first time in a long time that I did not have to put on a suit. I found my favorite pair of jeans and threw on a t-shirt.

Steve finished in the bathroom rather quickly. "Hey, I don't have to shave today," he said with a smile on his face.

"And I don't have to wear a suit today."

We high-fived, and I smacked him on his bare butt. As an avid powerlifter, Steve has what is called a "squat butt"—nicely shaped and very firm. Besides his biceps, it is my favorite part of his body.

"Where are we going for dinner?" I asked.

"What do you feel like eating? I could eat a horse. I'm starving," he responded.

With that response there was only one place in town: a pizzeria with homemade Italian food.

I walked over to my nightstand and put on my gun and badge. Besides Steve's presence, it was the only other thing that made me feel safe. I grabbed a jacket and threw it on for cover.

The pizza place was around the corner, and when we pulled into the lot, it was packed. "I guess everyone else had the same idea," Steve said.

We walked into the restaurant and grabbed the only remaining table. I sat down and took a deep breath, savoring the smell of fresh bread, pizza, and garlic. I could almost taste the calzone I was going to have.

Steve went up to the counter to place our order as I sat quietly in the booth facing the front door. Chivalry would dictate that the man should take that seat, but law enforcement training dictated the opposite. I always kept an eye on who was coming through the front door.

The restaurant's television was on, and it faced my direction. News coverage of yesterday's events played over and over. As soon as they replayed footage of the people jumping, I started to sweat. My heart began racing, and I couldn't catch my breath. Right then Steve returned to the booth.

"Sam, are you okay? You're white as a sheet."

I took Steve's hand. "Can you please ask them to turn the television off?"

Steve swung his head around and looked at the television. "Oh, God," he muttered. "I'll be right back."

I sat there with my head in my hands, trying to breathe normally.

Steve walked to the counter. I heard him say "Excuse me, could you do me a really big favor?" They talked for about thirty seconds, and then the television screen went black. I found that I could breathe again. I turned to the employee and mouthed the words, "Thank you."

Our food came a few minutes later, and we dove right in. The smell of fresh garlic and pizza dough filled my senses. I leaned down, closed my eyes, and breathed in through my nose, taking it all in. I picked up my knife and fork and cut the calzone in half. The melted cheese and meat oozed out from the middle, mixing with the homemade sauce. I breathed deeply through my nose again. My mouth watered as I prepared to dive in.

I looked over at Steve. "I'd like to freeze this moment," I said, smiling.

He reached across the table and took my hand. "I love you, Sam."

"I love you, too. Thank you for being with me."

Steve smiled back.

The calzone was calling my name. It had cooled down to where I could start eating. A few minutes later it was gone. I hadn't realized how hungry I was. I finished before Steve.

I was a fast eater in general because of the nature of my job. "Eat, and eat fast, because you don't know when your next meal will come," my supervisor often said.

I sat back in the booth and waited for Steve to finish. We decided to take another walk to work off some of the high-calorie, dense deliciousness we had just consumed. Steve paid the bill, and we walked toward the door.

I stopped at the counter and thanked the employee again for turning off the TV. In response she said, "Thank you for what you did."

I paused. "You're welcome," I said.

Steve took my hand, and we left the restaurant and walked back to the car. The evening air now had a touch of humidity in it. Once back at my apartment, we decided to go for a walk. I took off my gun, handcuffs, and pager and put them on the nightstand. I changed into shorts and sneakers again, put my fanny pack on with my gun inside, and clipped my pager onto my shorts. Steve was already ready waiting in the kitchen. We strolled through the neighborhood, stopping to look at flowers and interesting plants along the way.

We returned to my apartment just as the sun was setting. The minute we hit my apartment door, the phone started to ring. Family checked in for the next hour or so. Steve watched television in the living room as I sat in the kitchen. I reassured everyone that I was fine. At eight-thirty I hung up the phone and joined Steve on the couch. He was watching ESPN's coverage of the previous Sunday's football games. After each game was covered, the sportscaster reported on whether or not games would be played the following Sunday. With all flights grounded, teams would not be able to travel. The following day, September 13, 2001, the NFL commissioner decided to cancel all Week Two football games.

It seemed as though everything had been affected by the attack. The roads were closed, phone service was spotty, all airline travel came to a halt, and we had no field office. Steve and I sat in silence on the couch listening to the NFL commissioner lay out plans for the remainder of the season when my pager sounded.

The message outlined our squad meeting at ten the next morning at JFK. With several of the roads into and around the city closed to traffic, we were advised of approved routes, depending on where we lived. I knew from the route I was to take that Steve and I would need an hour and a half in the morning to get there on time (which meant at least ten to fifteen minutes before the scheduled start time).

At ten o'clock we decided to turn in. I was nervous about the morning, not sure how Steve would be received. I tried to concentrate on sleep. Desperately feeling worn out, I set the alarm for the next day, curled up next to Steve and fell asleep.

In the middle of the night Steve shook me awake.

"What is going on?" I asked. I had a dim recollection of him lying on top of me.

"You were having a nightmare."

Then came a flash followed by a loud boom. I instinctively dove under Steve.

"What is that?" I yelled.

"Sam, it's thunder. You're okay. I'm here."

"What is going on?"

"You were having a dream, Sam," Steve said. "You were trying to get underneath me."

Then it came again. *Boom!*

"Make it stop! Make it stop!" I yelled.

"Sam, I'm right here. You're safe. You're fine," Steve said as he helped me sit up. He took my head in his hands and looked into my eyes. "Sam, you are safe."

The storm moved quickly through the area until all that remained were faint flashes of lightning.

I looked over at the clock. Four-fifteen. Exasperated, I had no idea how I was going to fall back asleep. My heart was racing, and I was completely soaked in sweat. I got up and went to the bathroom. I splashed water on my face, and as I dried it, I looked into the mirror. *Sam, what the hell is going on with you?*

As a child I could vividly remember a recurring dream I had involving a snake, but this was different. I was transported right back to being in the elevator, followed by seeing the jumpers and the buildings crumbling right before my eyes.

I walked back into the bedroom and changed into dry pajamas. I climbed back into bed, and Steve held me.

"Do you want to talk about it?" he asked.

"I don't know how to make sense of it," I responded. "I saw everything that happened yesterday. The people jumping, the towers coming down. You said I was trying to get underneath you?"

"Yes. You were screaming, 'No, no. Not again,'" he said.

"I don't know. I'm all confused," I replied.

"Let's just try and get some more sleep."

FOUR

THE DEBRIEFING

"GOOD MORNING. IT'S a beautiful day in New Jersey. You're listening to 105.7, The Hawk." I reached over and turned off the alarm on my clock radio.

"Is it time already?" I said. I rolled over and tried to get out of bed. I felt exhausted, and it was if I had two concrete shoes on my feet. "Getting coffee," I muttered to Steve.

I walked into the kitchen to start my daily caffeine ritual. As I downed my first cup, Steve quietly walked into the kitchen and put his arms around me while I stared out the window trying to catch a glimpse of what the storm left behind in its wake. A few scattered tree limbs and leaves lay in the parking lot.

"Good morning," Steve whispered in my ear. Then he kissed me on my cheek.

"Morning," I said, kissing the arm that was wrapped around my shoulder.

We stood there for a few minutes. A bird landed on the windowsill and stared at us. We watched as it cocked its head back and forth as if it was trying to figure us out. When it flew away, Steve kissed me on the other cheek. "Breakfast time," he said. He got right to work making his breakfast.

"I'll take mine in the car when we leave," I said, filling my coffee mug up a second time with fresh coffee.

I went into the bathroom and started the shower. I kept the door open, as well as a portion of the shower curtain. As the hot water streamed down over my face, I closed my eyes. I could not block out the image of a man I watched jump to his death. My heart started to race, and I opened my eyes. I stood in the shower for a while trying to make sense of the nightmare, the storm, the images I kept seeing.

I finished my shower, walked into the bedroom, and stared at my closet. I should have been dressing for diplomatic meetings for the United Nations event. Instead I put on my favorite pair of jeans, which smelled like last night's delicious dinner, a sweatshirt, and my sneakers. I returned to the kitchen to refresh my mug of coffee. Steve had finished his breakfast, and we hugged each other. His big teddy bear-like embrace felt so safe and comforting—I had no idea how much I would come to rely on it.

When Steve was ready, we got into his car and made our way to the turnpike. As Steve drove we both noticed how few cars we saw. The local roads on the way to the turnpike should have been crowded already with people commuting to work. The commuters were replaced with law enforcement vehicles, both marked and unmarked. They seemed to be on every other street corner. Driving a black BMW convertible with Maryland tags, we definitely stuck out.

As we made our way to the airport, I started feeling uneasy. My head started to pound, and I fought back tears. I turned and looked out the window—I didn't want Steve to see my tears. I

THE DEBRIEFING

turned on the radio and focused on the music, hoping to take my mind off the debriefing to come.

When we pulled onto the airport service grounds, we were stopped by the Port Authority police. I presented my law enforcement credentials and Steve showed his driver's license. We were permitted to pass and pulled into the parking lot of one of the General Aviation Services buildings. I took a deep breath to try and release some of the stress.

"Ready?" Steve asked.

"Not really. But I don't have much of a choice, do I?"

My supervisor met us outside. "Hey, Sam. Good to see you. How are you doing?"

"Um, I'm okay, I guess. It's good to see everyone," I replied. "This is Steve. I appreciate you letting him bring me out."

"Hey, Steve, glad to meet you," my supervisor said as he shook Steve's hand. "Thanks for taking care of our girl here."

"It's an honor, sir. I'm very sorry about what happened to you guys. I was born in Brooklyn and grew up right across the George Washington Bridge in Jersey, so this is personal for me."

"Well, it's good to have you here with us then. We'll need to check you in and have you sign some papers. We will be sharing confidential information, and we'll need you to sign off indicating you won't reveal any of it," he replied.

We walked in to the building. Steve went with my supervisor, as I walked over to where some of my squad mates were standing.

"Hey, guys," I said.

"Hey, Sam. We were just talking about that storm last night," one of my squad mates said.

"Oh my gosh, it was insanely loud," I said. I didn't dare reveal what happened to me, but I knew my experience was not the only one. Silence fell between us as we looked at each other and then down at the floor. Steve walked over to the group.

"Guys, I'd like you to meet my boyfriend, Steve. He drove up Tuesday night from Maryland after the New Jersey guys dropped me off."

One by one my squad mates shook Steve's hand and introduced themselves.

"You don't live in Jersey?" one of my squad mates asked.

"Used to. I was born in Brooklyn and grew up in Bergen County, just across the bridge. I've been in Maryland for a while. That's where Sam and I met," Steve replied.

"That's cool, man. Good to have you with us."

"Thanks. I appreciate you guys letting me be here to support Sam. I'm sorry you had to go through what you did. I know it was tough. Everyone in DC is thinking about you guys up here—so just know you are not alone," Steve said, looking right into the eyes of one of my squad mates.

I couldn't help but feel a sense of pride. Here's a guy who couldn't be further removed from the United States Secret Service, and he's being accepted by my squad mates.

"Okay, folks, listen up," said the assistant to the special agent in charge (the ATSAIC). "We're going to get started with a roll call, and then you are going to split up by squad and report to the following rooms. Credit Cards will be in room one. Counterfeit in room two, TSD in room three, Electronic Crimes room four . . ." The list went on until each squad was assigned a room. "Grab some coffee or water, respond when you hear your name, and then report to your assigned room."

THE DEBRIEFING

As the ATSAIC called each agent's name, a few in my squad were noticeably missing.

"Anyone seen the folks who did not respond?" the ATSAIC asked after he was through.

A few people responded affirmatively, and my ATSAIC called them over. The rest of us went to our assigned rooms. Steve and I walked into room four, where the room had been set up with the chairs in a big circle. There were two women that I didn't recognize.

"Come on in and a take a seat," one of them said.

We filed in and slowly took our seats. Our supervisors came in after us and sat down. It felt strange because they were usually the ones leading the briefings.

"Hello, everyone. My name is Beverly, and this is my co-worker Susan. We're from Human Resources in DC. We've been sent from headquarters to help you guys out. Susan and I are assigned to the Safety and Health Division."

We all looked at each other from around the room, silently trying to figure out which division she was referring to.

"During your application process, you would have met with one of our staff who would have administered the psychological battery."

Oh, I thought to myself, *the head shrinkers.* I looked around the room and knew I wasn't the only one who silently had put two and two together. Some people moved uncomfortably in their chairs.

"Don't worry," said Beverly. "We know what you're thinking, and there's nothing going into anyone's file. We're here to help you walk through Tuesday's events. We've been doing this for more than twenty years, and when a traumatic event happens like it did to you folks, it helps to talk it out. We realize it will be harder for some of you than others, and that's okay. I'll start."

She paused and said, "Hi, I'm Beverly, and on April 15, 1995, I was in the Alfred P. Murrah Federal Building in Oklahoma City when it was bombed."

We all looked up at Beverly and nodded our heads as if to say, "Okay, Beverly, you can be in our club." Six Secret Service agents had died there, too.

Beverly went on to explain that she needed us to tell her where we were when the planes hit and where we were when the towers collapsed. She instructed us to take our time.

One by one we went around the circle and shared our accounts. One agent told of having to dive under a fire truck to avoid the falling debris. Another picked up a trashcan and smashed a storefront window, jumping inside before the twisted metal and dust cloud could reach him. A third commandeered a street vendor's hot-dog cart and pulled it into an alley where he used it as a shield against the falling debris.

When it was time for me to give my account, I choked up. I opened my mouth, but the only thing that came out were squeaks as I tried to hold back the tears. I put my finger in the air and motioned for Beverly to give me a minute. I took a few sips of water to regain my composure. Steve squeezed my hand tightly. Every time I started to speak, I could feel the dust in the back of my throat and coughed to try and clear my throat. I sipped more water. Finally I was able to speak.

"I was in the elevator in Tower One with several people. The elevator shook and the lights flickered. I thought we were getting stuck. Then came a noise I can't describe, and the next thing I knew the elevator was moving fast, and then it stopped. The doors flew open and hot air and dust smacked me in the face. Papers were flying everywhere. I watched a security guard spin in circles. Something was telling me there was a bomb and that I needed to get out. I grabbed a pregnant woman in the elevator, and we went up the escalator and out the exit door. Stuff was falling everywhere. I looked up and saw a man with a red tie leaning out of the building waving a white towel or something."

Beverly interjected. "Where were you when the towers fell?"

I looked at her with a puzzled expression. I thought she wanted to know where we were and what happened—why was she interrupting me? I paused and then answered, "I ran into the high school with the other agents when Tower Two came down, and I was on West Side Highway when Tower One collapsed. Kathy and Paul were with me. We were carrying a student, and when the tower came down, we ran as fast as we could with him. We passed him off to an ambulance crew that had stopped for us."

I looked up at Beverly, who had a pained expression on her face. "I met up with the rest of the agents at Pier 63 as instructed after that."

I let out a sigh of relief, and Steve patted my knee. I was sweating bullets. Some of my fellow agents were starting to cough. We continued our debriefing. Patrick, one of the youngest and newest agents in our squad, was caught in the collapse. He shared that a firefighter pulled him behind his truck to shield him from the debris hitting the truck like bullets. When he told us he thought he was going to die, we all lost it. There wasn't a dry eye in the room. Patrick said what we had all been thinking at some point that day.

When we were through, Beverly and Susan thanked us for being vulnerable and brave. They passed out their business cards and told us we could call them any time if we needed help. We sat there, dazed and confused, overwhelmed with everything we heard and shared.

Our supervisor entered the room. I could tell by his facial expression he was about to tell us something we did not want to hear.

"I know today was tough for all of you, and I appreciate you coming together to talk. It makes me sad to report that we suffered a loss on Tuesday," he began.

We looked around at each other, thinking the worst—that one of our squad mates had been killed. He broke the news that one of the support staff from DC assigned to the armored vehicles was missing and feared dead. His wife had been notified.

"Did he have any kids?" one of the agents asked.

"Yes," our supervisor said, looking down at the floor to hide the tears in his eyes.

We looked around the room at each other. Some of the agents who had children covered their faces so no one could see them cry. Others left the room. It was so quiet you could hear a pin drop.

"Don't any of you worry," the supervisor said. "His wife and kids will be taken care of. That's what we do."

On the day of his memorial service (none of his remains were recovered), it was standing room only at St. Elizabeth's Catholic Church. The NYPD covered us by maintaining a security zone several blocks out. The director, deputy director, and many others at the top came in from DC to attend. They also surprised each of us in the New York Field Office with Directors Citations for our heroic actions. None of us were in the mood to accept the citations. Being called heroes made us all feel guilty—there was so much more we could have done. A year later I would learn that this guilt is called "survivor's guilt."

"All right everyone, bring it in," our SAIC (Special Agent In Charge) said. We filed out of the room into the main area. "We just got word that POTUS is coming in tomorrow. He's going to Ground Zero." There was an exasperated response around the room. With everything that just happened to us, how were we as a field office going to handle a visit from the president? We had no resources. Everything had been destroyed when our building came down. There was mumbling and side conversations.

"Okay, people. I know what you're thinking. Quiet down," he said. "We are pulling in all the agents from New Jersey, Boston, and Pennsylvania to work this detail. For those of you that have your gun, badge, and handcuffs, you can volunteer to work the detail. Look, we do not expect you to work if you do not want to. This is a volunteer assignment."

A few agents raised their hands to volunteer. "If you want to work, get with your supervisors so we can get final numbers."

I walked outside with Steve. He asked if I was going to volunteer, and I said no. I needed to get home to see my mom. I always volunteered for historic assignments, but this was different. The attack was personal, and I was having a hard time focusing on any one thing for a long period of time. I was not 100 percent, and an agent running on less than 100 percent meant the potential that something could go unnoticed.

I found my supervisor and explained that while I wanted to volunteer, I simply could not. I needed to go home and be with my family for a few days. He understood and told me to inform him of my return date.

I could not look at him during our conversation—I felt like I was letting him down. He reached out and touched my shoulder. "Hey, Sam. It's okay. No one is going to say anything about it. We're all hurting," he said.

"Okay, thanks. Almost everyone in this field office has family here. I don't; my entire support system is in Maryland," I said.

"I understand," he said with concern in his eyes. "Go be with your family."

He turned to Steve. "Make sure she gets to her family, okay?"

"Yes, sir. I will," Steve responded.

We turned to walk to Steve's car. "My supervisor called to me, and I turned around. "I almost forgot," he said. "Headquarters wants everyone to get chest X-rays." He explained that everyone who was close to the building collapses has to get a chest X-ray because of all the asbestos and crap that we inhaled. He instructed me to stop by any clinic before I left and call him with the name of the clinic and the cost.

After getting into Steve's car, I grabbed my cell phone and called Information. I had no idea where I was going to get a chest X-ray. Information was able to connect me with a small clinic just north of Newark. I called the clinic to find out what exit off the turnpike we should take, and we arrived thirty minutes later. Steve found a parking space in the shade.

THE DEBRIEFING

"Ready?" Steve asked.

I grabbed him and pulled him close. The tears began to flow uncontrollably. The impact of all of the close calls my squad mates shared had hit me full force, and I needed an outlet. Steve held me close until I was able to regain my composure.

"I'm good now," I said.

Steve reached out and touched my chin. I looked up at him.

"Really, I'm okay now. Sorry," I said, wiping my eyes.

"Why are you apologizing, Sam? Come here," Steve said as he pulled me close. We held each other. I felt safe, and I knew he would not let anything happen to me.

I broke the embrace and took his hand. We walked into the clinic. Steve took a seat, and I went to the front desk.

"Hi, I'm Agent Perper. I called a few minutes ago about a chest X-ray."

"Oh, yes. Secret Service, right? That's so cool," the receptionist said.

I looked around the waiting room to see who may have overheard her say "Secret Service." It was not something I wanted broadcast. We were trained to be seen but unseen, depending on the circumstances, so we had the element of surprise. It was easier for the female agents to do this, because most people assumed that all Secret Service agents were tall males wearing dark suits and sunglasses and running next to the president's limousine. Most of the public had no idea about the major criminal investigations we were involved in or that the majority of the time we wore plainclothes. We made it a point to blend in, whether we were shopping for groceries, at the movies, or attending sporting events. Most had no idea there was a highly skilled law enforcement officer anywhere near them.

She handed me a stack of forms to fill out before I could get the X-ray.

"Wow, that's a lot of forms. Do you need to know what color underwear I'm wearing?" I said to her. It was a small attempt at humor that she missed.

I completed the forms ten minutes later and returned to the front desk. "I want to point out that the address for workman's comp is a Washington, DC, address—our headquarters. We don't have a field office anymore," I said.

The front desk woman looked up at me, puzzled.

"Our Field Office was in 7 World Trade Center. It was the last building to come down on Tuesday."

"Oh, yes, I understand now," she said. "I'm sorry."

Someone opened the main door to the office area. "Samantha?" she said. "I'm Sarah. I'm going to take your X-rays today." I followed her into the X-ray room. I looked around the room as Sarah read the forms.

"Oh, wow," she said. "You were there on Tuesday. Thank you for your service."

"You're welcome," I responded.

An awkward silence followed. Finally she said, "May I ask you a question?"

"Sure," I responded.

"What was it like on Tuesday?"

I looked down at the floor, trying to come up with an answer.

"I'm sorry," she said. "You don't have to answer that."

I looked up at her. "No, it's okay. Think about your favorite action movie. Where the good guy is in a shootout with or taking out the bad guy. Put yourself in the scene as the good guy."

"Okay," she said.

"Now imagine you've got things exploding all around you, and you know there's a bad guy you have to take out, but he's nowhere to be found. You're running around with your gun drawn, trying to figure out who is causing this mess, but no matter which direction you run, there's nothing but more bodies and more debris falling from the sky. That's what it was like."

"Oh my gosh, that's crazy," she said.

A few minutes later we were finished. We walked back down the hall. "The report will be ready in a few days and sent to the Washington, DC, address. I'm not supposed to say but everything looks clear," the technician said.

"Thank you," I said as I shook her hand.

"No, thank you."

I smiled and met up with Steve back in the waiting room.

"Let's go," I said.

Walking back to the car, we decided that food was necessary and next on the agenda.

"Let's get out of here," Steve said, pulling his door closed.

We started back to the turnpike. I recommended taking the local roads so we could find the closest restaurant. I also had no idea if we were going to be able to get on the turnpike.

"What about calling your parents to see if they want to have dinner with us?" I said.

"Great idea," he said as picked up his phone. We decided on Empire Hunan, a favorite of ours. I could practically taste the spare ribs; they were the best outside of Chinatown.

The X-ray technician's report that my X-ray was clear perked my spirits, and I was looking forward to spending an evening out. Steve and I got a table in the far corner and waited for his parents to arrive. The waiter took our drink order. When Steve's parents arrived, we ordered another round to go with our orders of spare ribs. Dinner arrived a few minutes later.

"So, Sam, how are you doing? We were so scared on Tuesday," Steve's mom said.

"I'm doing okay," I said, lying through my teeth. I didn't tell them about the thunderstorm or not being able to close the bathroom door. "It's great to have Steve here."

"What are you going to do now?" Steve's dad asked.

"Steve is driving me back to Maryland. I'm going to spend some time with my mom and see my family."

"We can only imagine what it was like on Tuesday. When you get back up here, please let us know if we can do anything," Steve's mom said.

"Thanks, I will." I motioned for the waiter to bring me another drink. It was the only thing allowing me to talk about Tuesday.

He put the third bottle down on the table. Steve reached over and grabbed my hand before I could pick it up. Silently he was asking if I was okay.

"Sam, we can understand if you don't want to talk about it. But if you don't mind, can you tell us what happened to you?" I looked over at Steve's mom and took a long sip of my drink.

"Mom, I think Sam's had enough today," Steve said, protecting me.

"No, it's okay, Steve. People want to know." I took another long sip of my drink.

THE DEBRIEFING

I asked them if they had watched any of the television coverage, and they both responded that they had.

"Well, imagine yourself right there, experiencing everything you watched on TV in surround sound turned up so loud that that your brain is screaming, but there's nothing you can do so you just continue to move, trying to stay alive."

Steve's parents shifted uncomfortably in their chairs, unable to respond. A palpable silence fell across our table, was broken by the waiter who came to the table with the check.

"Okay, we've all had a long day, so let's call it a night. We have to be on the road early tomorrow," Steve said. We got up from the table and gave each other hugs good-bye.

As we got into the car, Steve said, "Sam, are you okay? Your response to my parent's question was a little abrupt."

"I guess I'm just a little stressed. It's been a crazy day, and it all kind of hit me at one time. I'm sorry. I'll call them tomorrow and apologize," I said.

Steve reached over and squeezed my hand. I looked over at him, took his face in my hands, and kissed him gently. "I love you," I said.

"I love you, too," he whispered.

We didn't talk much on the way back to my apartment. I was feeling angry—it had started over dinner. I did not know how to shut it off, so I just stayed quiet.

FIVE

WARNING SIGNS

WHEN WE GOT home, packing for the trip back to Maryland was my first priority. While Steve made a few business calls and watched television, I grabbed a beer and disappeared into the bedroom where I kept my luggage. There was one full suitcase and one empty one already on the floor in my closet. This was part of an agent's repertoire: one bag always ready to go next to the one you just returned with because sometimes there were only a few hours in between assignments. I threw some clothes into the empty bag, returned to the kitchen for another beer, and plopped down on the couch next to Steve. The alcohol took the edge off, and I was starting to feel relaxed. I couldn't remember the last time I was able to have multiple drinks on a weeknight. But since I was not going to be on duty for a while, I figured why not.

Before long I started to drift off to sleep. Steve woke me up. "C'mon Sam. Let's go to bed." He took my hand and led me to the bedroom, where I quickly changed and then went into the bathroom to wash up. I returned to the bedroom and crawled into bed. The blankets felt so good as I scrunched them up underneath me. I was asleep before Steve got into bed.

"Sam, wake up!" Steve said as he shook me.

"What? What's going on?" I said groggily.

"You were having another dream."

"Oh no," I said, putting my hand on my head.

"I'm sorry for waking you." It was 4:15 a.m. "Do you remember what you were dreaming about?"

"Not really. It's all kind of jumbled in my head. I remember the jumper."

On September 11th there were many things that bombarded my brain. The most disturbing were the people who consciously jumped to their death rather than being burned to death. Being only two blocks away, I had a clear view of them. There was one in particular that I dubbed "the jumper"—I followed him from the moment I saw him falling through the air until he hit the pavement; I felt the shockwaves. He was wearing a dark suit with a red tie. The tie trailed behind him as he fell.

Steve pulled me close to him and I dozed off again until 8:00 a.m. when my alarm went off.

"Coffee," I said as I dragged myself out of bed and into the kitchen. I poured myself my first cup and headed to the bathroom. I was anxious to get on the road. I quickly showered and dressed and was ready to go by 9:30 a.m. I poured the last of the coffee in my travel mug as Steve loaded our bags in the car. I locked my apartment door and headed downstairs where Steve was already waiting.

"I see you want to get back, too," I said.

"It'll be good to be with everyone for a few days. I have to get back to work, but we'll definitely get together every night."

I leaned over and kissed Steve. "Thank you," I said.

"You don't have to thank me. But you're welcome," he said, smiling back at me.

WARNING SIGNS

We pulled out of my apartment complex, made a few quick turns, and turned onto the New Jersey Turnpike South. Just as earlier in the week, the roads were empty. We stopped once along the way and made it to my mom's house in record time. We pulled into her driveway, and she ran out the front door to meet me. She wrapped her arms around me. "Oh, my baby, my sweet baby," she cried.

We stayed in the driveway. I closed my eyes and savored being wrapped in the best-ever mom hug. When I opened my eyes, I noticed that the neighbors were coming out of their homes. My mom lived in a very tight community where pretty much everyone knew each other. Everyone knew I was an agent assigned to the New York Field Office; everyone knew I worked at the World Trade Center. One by one they came over to say hello and hug me. I appreciated their kindness and support. After about thirty minutes I said my "see ya laters" and "thank yous" and disappeared into my mom's house. Steve followed with my luggage.

"That was really sweet of everyone, Mom," I said.

"We really have such a great community here. Everyone looks out for everyone," she responded. Turning to Steve and giving him a hug, she said, "I can't thank you enough for bringing my baby home."

"You're so welcome, Vicki. I'll let you guys be, and I'll see you tonight," he responded.

"Yes, please come at seven. Nan, Papa Harry, Lee, Gail, and Jorge are coming by so we can all be together." I smiled as I thought, *My mom, still the ultimate planner.* She always organized the family get-togethers when I came to town.

I walked into my old bedroom with my bag. I quickly

changed into my nightclothes and hugged my mom. "It's good to be home," I said.

"How are you, honey?" she asked, sounding concerned.

I explained that I was not sleeping well and felt worn out. I asked her to let me sleep and wake me an hour before dinner if necessary. I crawled beneath the cool sheets, pulled the blanket up over my head, and drifted off to sleep.

It was as if it were snowing outside. The sun was shining, but everything was gray. I looked up to the sun and it shone brightly back at me. *Boom!* The ground shook. I threw my hands out to steady myself. *Boom!* A fireball shot from the sky. I realized the snowflakes were ashes. I looked behind me and saw "the jumper." As if someone was fast-forwarding through a movie, I saw "the jumper" over and over again.

"No!" I yelled, sitting up in bed. I was soaked with sweat. I put my head in between my hands and took a deep breath. The nightmare had followed me home. "Damn it," I said to myself.

I heard scratching at my door—my miniature schnauzer Solomon wanted in. I opened the door, picked him up, and held him on my lap. I turned on the television. Sports was the only safe thing for me to watch, so I turned on ESPN's *Sports Center* and watched coverage of the NFL commissioner's press conference. He announced that all games were postponed for the weekend.

My mom came in the bedroom and sat down on the bed next to me and Solomon. "I couldn't really sleep," I said as I hugged my dog.

"Uncle Lee is on his way over with Gail," Mom said.

"Okay, I'll jump in the shower then." I put Solomon on the floor and made my way to the bathroom. After a quick shower (which I was now able to perform without leaving the door open and the shower curtain open), I joined my uncle and his wife, Gail, in the living room. I gave everyone a big hug. I noticed two bottles of wine on the dining room table. "Oh, yummy," I said, walking over to the wine.

"I thought you might like some, Sam. We got it at a festival—it's really good," Gail said, showing me the label.

"Let's open it," I said enthusiastically.

Mom handed me two wine glasses. Neither she nor Uncle Lee drank. I opened the bottle and poured the wine into each of our glasses. It was a nice pouring cabernet. I swirled it in my glass, sniffed it, and then took a small sip. "Oh, that's nice," I said. It had a medium body to it. "This is definitely a keeper."

Less than an hour later, the first bottle was gone.

My grandparents arrived. Papa Harry was wearing a Secret Service cap. After graduating from the Academy, I had given it to him. He wore it everywhere; tonight was no exception.

"It's so good to see you guys," I said as I wrapped an arm around each of them. I let out a big sigh as I hugged them.

The door opened and Steve came in with the food—Chinese takeout from our family's favorite place. We'd been regular customers for more than five years. He also brought a bottle of wine his brother Robert recommended. Robert is a true wine connoisseur, with a collection of over a thousand bottles in his wine cellar in Kirkland, Washington, where he lives.

"Let's eat!" I said. The last meal I had was breakfast in the car, and I was famished.

We all gathered around and helped ourselves to the various dishes. I opened the bottle of wine Steve brought and sat down at the table my mom had set for all of us. It felt great to be with my family. Since we had already spoken on the phone on September 11th, we talked about anything and everything else. It was refreshing. The wine helped take the edge off, too.

By 9:30 p.m., our bellies full and all the wine drunk, we were ready to call it an evening. Steve, my aunt, and my uncle all had to work the next day. We all walked outside together. I promised to see them again before going back to New Jersey. Steve helped my grandparents into their car, and we saw everyone off. He and I waited until everyone left before saying our good night. We walked over to his car. I wrapped my arms around his neck, and he kissed me—long, passionate, and deep. "I love you, Sam," he said after we came up for air.

"I love you, too. I'll see you tomorrow." I watched Steve pull away and thought about how nice it would be to come home to someone each night. As soon as he rounded the corner, I walked back into my mom's house. She was in the kitchen cleaning up. I gave her a big hug and thanked her for having everyone over. The wine had taken full effect, and I was feeling tired.

"C'mon Solomon." I motioned for my dog to come in the bedroom with me. He followed quickly, and I picked him up and put him on the bed. He made a beeline for my pillow. "Hey fuzz-bucket, that's my pillow," I said. He gently licked me on the nose in response.

I turned on the TV and pulled the covers down. Between the wine and the mindless squawk box, I fell asleep in no time.

∽

The next morning I woke up still feeling tired, but I noticed I hadn't dreamt at all. *Hmm,* I thought. I wandered into the kitchen where my mom already had the coffee on for me.

"Hi, honey—seems like you slept well."

The coffeepot was near the clock in the kitchen. As I poured my cup, I looked up. The clock read 11:00 a.m. "Is that the right time?" I asked.

"Yes, it is."

"Holy crap, I guess I was tired!" I said. I turned to look out the side door off the kitchen. There was a bird's nest with three little baby birds chirping away. I walked over to take a closer look, coffee in hand. I closed my eyes, took a sip of my coffee, and enjoyed the sounds of the baby birds.

Boom! It came out of nowhere. The noise startled me so much that I spilled some of my coffee on my hand as I ducked for cover. "Damn it!" I yelled.

"Are you okay?" my mom called from the bedroom.

"Yeah—but what was that?"

"A dumpster truck," she said.

Why in the hell am I looking for cover from a dumpster truck? I thought.

I shook it off, poured myself some more coffee, and ran the hand the coffee burned under the cold water as I stared out the window at the leaves that had started to change for the fall season.

"What do you—"

"Holy crap, Mom!" I said as I jumped. "You scared me."

"I'm sorry, honey. I didn't mean to."

"I know. I'm sorry. What were you saying?" I asked.

I could see my mom's mouth moving, but I could not hear her

words. My heart was pounding, and I felt a surge of adrenaline rush through my body. My ears started to ring.

"Honey . . . Samantha. Are you okay?"

"I'm sorry, Mom. I'm just a little distracted," I said.

I couldn't tell my mom what was going on. I felt trapped in a very strange world filled with noises that penetrated my eardrums and caused reactions that were hasty and filled with anger.

"What do you want to do today?" Mom asked.

"Whatever you want is fine with me," I responded. I couldn't think of any better response because my brain simply felt as though it was on overload. My mom continued to talk, and I continued to pretend that I could hear what she was saying. I agreed to accompany her for the day.

Any normal, everyday activity would be a good idea, I thought. I got dressed and decided to leave my gun and handcuffs at home. Sam the Super Agent needed a break. I grabbed the keys to my mom's car.

"I'll wait for you in the car, Mom."

"Okay—I'll be right there, honey."

I kissed Solomon, patted him on the head, and walked out the door to my mom's car. She came out just after I closed the driver's side door.

"Where to?" I asked.

My mom looked at me strangely. "Samantha, I told you I had a doctor's appointment."

"Oh, yes, right. Let's go."

As we neared the doctor's office, I realized we were going to a familiar place. My mom's doctor had watched my sister and I grow up. As I turned into the parking lot, I started to feel uneasy. I really didn't feel like talking to anyone or pretending that everything was okay, but I didn't want my mom to think anything was wrong, so I put on my best face.

We entered the office, and I took a seat in the corner away from the television. I buried my face into one of those mindless magazines that occupies every doctor's office. My mom was called for her appointment, and about forty minutes later she came out. I met her at the check-out window.

"Marlene, you remember Samantha?" my mom said.

"Oh my goodness, Samantha. Your mom told me all about what you're doing. I'm so glad you got out of New York okay. What a terrible day! I can only imagine what you went through. I watched it on TV. Thank goodness you're with us."

As she spoke I found myself thinking, *Here we go again. Yes, you can only imagine . . .* I felt myself getting angry. For some reason I could not sympathize with what people must have seen through their television screens or the emotion they carried. My world was becoming smaller and more insulated by choice.

I thanked her for her kind words. "Mom, I'll meet you by the elevators," I said and walked out of the office.

"Where are we meeting Fran?" I asked once we were in the car. I happened to remember my mom mentioning her name before I "zoned out."

"Hamburger Hamlet," she said.

We didn't talk much on the way to the restaurant. We arrived at Hamburger Hamlet and walked inside, where Fran was waiting for us. She gave me a big hug. "Sam, it's so good to see you. Your mom and I talk every day. I'm so sorry you had to go through all of that."

"Thank you. I appreciate you checking in on Mom."

The hostess showed us to our table. "So how are you doing?" Fran asked. I know she meant well, but I was growing tired of talking about it.

"I'm okay. Staying away from all the news coverage—it's not like I don't know what happened. I'm catching up on a lot of missed sleep and enjoying being home," I responded.

We placed our order, and for the first time at lunch I ordered a beer. I normally only consumed alcohol in the evening, but I felt the need to take the edge off.

Lunch was relatively short because Fran had another appointment. "It was great seeing you, Sam. Thank you so much for your service and for what you did on 9/11. You helped so many people."

"Thank you. I was just doing my job."

We gave each other a hug and walked out to the car. Once inside I turned to my mom. "Mom, can we go home? I'm beat."

"Sure. I can do the rest of my errands later."

We drove home, and I immediately went into the bedroom and closed the door. I was irritated beyond words, and I couldn't figure out why. I had just turned on the television when I heard Solomon scratching on the door. I opened it, scooped up Solomon, and put him on my lap. At this point he was one of the few things that calmed me down. He looked up at me as if he knew what I needed and licked me on the chin. I flipped through the channels as I cradled him.

There was a knock at the door. "Honey, can I come in?" my mom asked.

I opened the door, and she sat on the end of the bed. "Honey, are you sure you're okay?" she asked.

"Why is everyone asking me that?" I exclaimed loudly.

My mom looked at me with a shocked expression on her face.

"Mom, I'm sorry. I'm not sure what's going on. Everything seems so loud. It's like I can't find any quiet."

"You've been through a very traumatic experience, sweetie. Sometimes strange things can happen to the brain."

I listened to what my mom said. I didn't want strange things to happen. I wanted to sleep; I wanted to work; I wanted to feel like myself again.

"What do you mean, strange things can happen to the brain?" I asked.

My mom went on to explain that when a traumatic event occurs, the brain goes into fight-or-flight as a protective mechanism. It becomes hypervigilant. Its overriding goal is to help you survive.

"But sometimes your brain can't shut down after the event. It releases hormones to help you deal with stress. I'd say your brain did a wonderful job the other day, honey."

I smiled.

"I think what's going on is that your brain is still releasing hormones because you are stressed. That's why you're tired and irritated."

"That makes sense," I said. "Will everything get back to normal again?"

"I don't know, honey. I'm pretty sure it will. You're a healthy person, so I don't see why not. You have to be patient."

Patience was not the word I wanted to hear. It was definitely one of the things I had to work on. When I was interviewed for any job and the interviewer asked, "What do you think one of your weaknesses is?" my response was always, "Patience." It never prevented me from getting the job, but it often stressed me out.

"Mom, I think I need to take all this in right now and try and get quiet," I said.

"I understand. I'll leave you and Solomon alone. I'm going to finish my errands." She left the room and closed the door behind her.

I turned to Solomon. "What do you think, Soli?" I kissed him on the head, curled up with him under the covers, and went to sleep.

A few hours later I awoke. Solomon was still curled up under the covers with me. I put him on the floor and walked into the kitchen were my mom was prepping for dinner.

"Hi, honey. Steve called—he's coming for dinner at seven."

I looked at the clock. It was almost six.

"Can you feed Soli and take him for a walk for me?" Mom asked.

"Absolutely," I responded, eager to get outside and move a little bit.

After feeding Soli, I walked outside and took a deep breath. There was a touch of humidity in the air. Solomon was eager to walk, and I followed behind. As we walked I made note of the leaves changing on the trees. There was one particular tree that stood out. Its leaves were red, yellow, and orange. The pattern of the leaves made it appear that the tree was on fire. It took me back to Ground Zero and the fires burning.

Solomon's barking snapped me out of my trance. I took a deep breath and continued my walk with Solomon. I savored the sunshine and the quiet time to walk and reflect on what occurred over the previous few days. I was playing with thanking God and cursing him at the same time—grateful I was still alive but confused over why he chose to allow 9/11 to happen in the first place. It was a naïve way to look at the situation.

I rounded the corner and headed back to the house. It was almost seven, and Steve would be arriving for dinner. My mom was putting the finishing touches on the dinner table. The aroma took me back to when I was a kid coming in from playing outside. Her chicken recipe had not changed; it was always something I looked forward to.

I took a deep breath in through my nose. "That smells so good," I said.

"I'm glad I could make it for you and Steve. I don't make it as much as I used to since it's just me."

"Well, I guess I'll have to visit more often then," I said with a smile.

There was a knock at the door. I let Steve in, kissed him hello, and then let him greet Solomon who was jumping up and down. Steve and Solomon had a welcome ritual I absolutely loved. Schnauzers are not known for howling, but Solomon loved to show off his voice. Steve got down on the floor, and Solomon put his front paws on his chest. Steve started to howl, and Solomon followed suit. My mom and I laughed.

The three of us sat down at the table for dinner. Steve had brought a bottle of wine to complement our meal.

"So I wanted to talk with you guys about the holidays, which start next week," my mom said.

The Jewish High Holidays were the holiest days of the year. Since becoming a Secret Service agent and moving to New Jersey,

I had stopped going to synagogue. An agent's life did not leave much room for religious worship since we worked so much. Now that I was taking time to be with family, I would have the opportunity go with my mom and grandmother to synagogue.

"I'll think about it, Mom," I said.

"Okay, honey. I'm not trying to put any pressure on you, but it would be nice for you to be with me and Nan."

In my mind I thought, *Oh-oh, here comes the guilt.*

We continued to eat, and I continued to drink—especially after the "guilt" my mom had just laid on me. We finished dinner a short time later.

"Do you want to go for a walk?" I asked Steve.

Solomon responded to the word *walk*. "Sure, let's go," Steve said.

I grabbed Solomon's leash, and we headed out the door. For whatever reason I felt the need to move my body. It was a strange feeling. One minute I was exhausted, and the next minute I wanted to move.

Steve took my hand, and we walked together as Solomon ran ahead of us. I was glad we could spend a few days together.

"Do you think you'll go to synagogue with your mom?" Steve asked.

"I don't know." I had so many different thoughts going through my head. I was pissed off at God that He let last Tuesday happen, but I was grateful to be alive.

"I'm grateful you're here, Sam. There must have been some plan from the Big Man upstairs, so whatever you decide, I'm sure it's the right decision."

We continued to walk quietly together. We said good-night

when we got back to my mom's house, and I walked inside with Solomon.

"Where's Steve?" my mom asked.

"He went home. He's got to see some patients tomorrow," I responded. I walked over to my mom and hugged her. "I'll let you know about the holidays soon, okay, Mom?"

"All right, honey. No problem. I love you."

"Love you, too, Mom."

That uneasy nighttime feeling started to return, and I needed something to take the edge off. I went into the kitchen where I found the leftover wine from dinner. I took the bottle and my glass to my bedroom and closed the door. I changed for bed, turned on a movie, and let the wine do its thing. Hopeful that it would prevent me from dreaming.

At three in the morning I woke up; the TV was still on. I turned it off, walked into the bathroom, and splashed some water on my face. As I looked in the mirror, I noticed the dark circles under my eyes. I walked back to the bedroom and crawled under the covers. Seven hours later I woke up to Solomon barking; I felt like a truck had run over me. I wandered out into the kitchen and made coffee immediately. Mom was not at home; her car wasn't in the driveway. I relished the quiet and not having to talk to anyone.

Thirty minutes later I started to feel better. I watched two hummingbirds at the feeder outside the kitchen. *I'd love to fly off with them,* I thought. With each passing day I became more and more uncomfortable in my own skin, and I didn't know what to do. The one thing I found comfort in was the fact that I could drink my nightmares away. I didn't realize it was a solution that would take me down a dark path.

My mom came home a few hours later. I was still in my pajamas.

"You're not dressed yet?" she said, looking at her watch.

"I'm just tired, Mom. I don't have anywhere to be, so . . ."

"Well then, you just do what you'd like today," she said with a certain disapproving tone.

I could tell she was not happy with me being in my pajamas this late in the afternoon. It was like I was back in high school. It had annoyed my mom no end when I stayed out late Saturday night and lounged around all day Sunday.

But this time being in my pajamas had nothing to do with being a lazy teenager. Most people, including my mom, had no idea of the stress and exhaustion that came with being a Secret Service agent. With some assignments allowing for only a few hours of sleep a night coupled with not the greatest of eating habits, it eventually caught up with you. I can remember a Snickers bar and a Coke being dinner on more than one occasion. Several of the agents nicknamed it "the dinner of champions." When it did catch up with you, there was zero motivation to do anything except rest. This was one of those days.

The next day I made my decision to attend High Holiday Services with my mom and my grandmother. When I told my mom, she was ecstatic. She confessed that she had telephoned the rabbi, told him I was coming, and arranged for me to be recognized during the service. When I found out, I was anything but excited. I just wanted to be left alone. I didn't feel like a hero. I had feelings of guilt. My mind kept telling me I could have saved more lives on September 11th, even though in reality I knew it was not possible. But I mustered up some excitement, acted surprised, and gave my mom a big hug. I wasn't going to ruin her proud moment.

When the time came to attend services a few days later, I put on my best face, smiled, shook a lot of hands, and said thank you over and over. When the rabbi gave his sermon, I listened attentively. When he said the words, "God loves everyone, regardless of who they are and what they've done," I lost it. I cried on my grandmother's shoulder.

The words didn't make sense to me. How could God love us when He just let more than two thousand people die? How could God love us when He gave people a choice to burn to death or jump to their deaths? And how on earth could God love those evil men who perpetrated the second worst attack on U.S. soil? At that moment I felt my heart turn to stone. I wanted out of the synagogue—I did not want to hear another word about how God supposedly loved us. This split-second decision led me down a path of personal destruction and loss. I closed the door to God—and to my heart.

"I'll meet you outside," I whispered to my mom. I got up from my seat and left the sanctuary. I went downstairs to the bathroom. All I felt was anger. Alone in the bathroom I looked at myself in the mirror. *You're not fooling me, God.* I thought.

My ego took over, and my expression changed. The "hero" now became the "villain"; a sense of darkness took hold of me. Everyone was the enemy—untrustworthy until proven otherwise. I did not want to hear about God or love or peace. We were at war, and as President Bush said at the time, "You are either with us or against us." I had no time nor the desire to debate with anyone about whether we should have gone to war. All I knew was that Mohammad Atta and his buddies tried to take me out, so I was going to shut the door to anyone who dared say anything about the war we were fighting being wrong.

I felt that the only people who "got me" and understood where I was coming from were my Uncle Lee, my grandparents, and Steve. I wanted to be with them as much as possible. I contacted my supervisor and let him know I'd be back to work in a few days. Soldier Sam was ready to do battle with anyone and anything.

SIX

BACK TO WORK

ON SUNDAY I said my good-byes, and Steve drove me to the train station. I arrived in New Jersey three hours later, hailed a cab, and returned to my apartment. I emptied my mailbox, which was stuffed with mail. Now I had to figure out how to get to my office. Where *was* my office?

I called Wilson, one of the senior agents in my squad. "Hey, it's Sam. I'm ready to dive back in. I've got a favor to ask . . ."

He knew exactly what I was going to ask. "I'll pick you up tomorrow at eight. We got some G-rides from other field offices. The guys in Boston sent one down for you. It's at the office."

"And where would that be now?"

Wilson laughed. He explained that our squad had rented space above a BMW dealership on the Upper West Side.

"So we get to drool at all the new cars as we go to work each morning. The best part is there's the greatest pizza place right up the street! The squads are spread out all over the city."

He continued to explain that the Credit Card squad was moving into the office space next to ours, and all hands on deck were needed to reprogram the computers, load the software, and grab all kinds of computer stuff from Staples. "Glad you're back to help, Sam."

"It feels great to be back. I'm here to help with anything and everything."

"Well, you better get some rest then. We're running 24/7 till everything's back online."

"Will do, Wilson. Thanks. See you in the morning."

I turned on the football game and prepped for tomorrow, making sure I had all of my equipment. As the evening went on, I started to feel anxious. This was the first time I was alone in over a week. I went to the fridge and opened it. I was happy to see a cold six-pack.

I opened the cabinet next to the fridge and saw an unopened bottle of wine. *Beer or wine?* I thought. I went with wine. I also cooked up some dinner. I planted myself in front of the television, and before I knew it the bottle was gone. I felt relaxed and ready to sleep.

At 6:00 a.m. the next morning, I awoke to my alarm clock. I felt surprisingly well, having slept through the night, no nightmares or restlessness. *Must have been the wine,* I thought.

I grabbed some coffee, did a short workout, and then jumped in the shower. By eight I was downstairs, coffee and bagel in hand. Wilson pulled into the parking lot, and I jumped in his new hand-me-down G-ride: a silver Chevy Lumina with a red velour interior.

"Nice ride," I said.

"Thanks. Full light package already installed," he replied.

"Now that's what I call a hand-me-down!" I exclaimed.

"No kidding. I was surprised when I got it."

As Wilson drove he filled me in on what was going on in our new location and our two new assignments. The first was the Joint Terrorism Task Force (JTTF). In the short time I was away, the president had ordered that all federal law enforcement agencies and their local counterparts be activated to form a task force to investigate terrorist activity. The was to assign one to two agents on a rotating basis until further notice. The JTTF Coordination Center was located at LaGuardia Airport.

The second assignment was at Fresh Kills, a large landfill on Staten Island, New York. Debris from Ground Zero was being brought there, where it was sorted through in order to recover human remains, personal effects, and evidence. This was a volunteer assignment made up of law enforcement personnel and forensic evidence specialists.

We exited at 14C for the Holland Tunnel. A sign read Law Enforcement and Emergency Services Vehicles Only. Wilson stopped at the checkpoint, and we both showed the Port Authority officer our credentials. He waved us through, and we zipped through the Holland Tunnel like never before. I could feel my heart pounding inside my chest as we emerged on the other side. Smoke still filled the air, and there was an odor of burning concrete. I took a deep breath to try and calm myself down. The smell brought me back . . .

We turned onto the West Side Highway. That's when I saw the freezer trucks lined up in the far right lanes. The smell of burning concrete grew stronger. I knew immediately what the freezer trucks were for. I started to feel nauseous. I had not heard of many bodies being recovered intact. I could only imagine the grief felt by the families who were hoping for some small miracle or confirmation with the recovery of remains.

We reached our new office building and parked in the back. There were several spaces that had yellow Xs across them.

"If you can find a space in the morning, park in one of these spots with the X and place your police placard in the dash," Wilson explained.

The police placard issued to every agent allowed our vehicles to be identified so we would not be towed or issued a ticket. There were only two rules: Don't block a fire hydrant, and don't park in a loading zone if possible.

We walked in through the back door. New BMW Mini Coopers were on display in the lobby.

"Nice," I said as we rounded the corner to the elevators. We got off on the third floor, where I noticed wires running everywhere. I followed Wilson into the open area ahead of us. *No doors?* I wondered.

"Look who I found!" Wilson exclaimed.

"Hi, Sam. Welcome back!" said CJ and Don.

"Hey, guys. Wow! What a setup," I replied as I looked around. There was stuff everywhere: binders piled in the corners with computer bags; more wire and huge dry-erase boards on rollers; six-foot folding tables being used as desks. I turned and saw a whiteboard in the corner with photos of the terrorists responsible for the 9/11 attacks. As I stood and stared, Don came up behind me.

"We're being asked to trace the money," he said. "Come on. I'll show you your desk." I followed Don into the next room. Two six-foot tables had been put together in an L shape.

"Here ya go, Sam. Go grab a laptop from the other room. Mark will give you the cables to go with it."

I was glad to hear Mark's name. He was one of the agents who went MIA after being ferried across to New Jersey on 9/11. He was also an IT expert who had come from the computer industry before joining the Secret Service."

"Hey, Mark. Great to see you."

"Hi, Sam. It's good to be seen. Come on over. I'm almost finished loading the software on this one so you can have it."

The room was filled with more than fifty IBM ThinkPads.

"Cool. Thanks." I looked around. The CD/DVD drives were open on almost all of the laptops. Mark went around to each and put disks in the trays.

"Where'd all these laptops come from?" I asked.

"Ben called IBM, and they gave them to us."

"That's cool. Is there anyone Ben doesn't know?"

"I know, right?" Mark said with a laugh.

Mark asked if I could help him load the software. Like him, I had not been a law enforcement officer prior to being hired by the Secret Service, and I knew my way around basic computer software and hardware.

"Sure, let me ask Don." I walked into the other office where Don was sitting and asked if I could help Mark with the computers.

"Oh my gosh, Sam, I totally forgot you had those skills! Get your butt in there—we needed those laptops yesterday," he exclaimed with a smile.

I smiled back. Everything I knew about computers was self-taught. I was no expert, but I could navigate through the computer prompts with ease. I walked back to Mark's office Mark. "I'm all yours."

"Thanks, Sam. Here's your machine. Put a sticky note on it so it doesn't grow legs."

Mark proceeded to tell me what programs needed to be loaded

and the particular sequence I needed to follow. The stacks of CDs were next to each machine. Some were labeled, while others were not.

"Keep loading the CDs until you see the disc with the number one on it. That means all programs have been loaded and it's ready to go. If there's a machine that can't read the disc, take it off the table and put it over there." He pointed to the far corner where there were already several laptops stacked up.

"Got it," I responded. I went to work.

We worked in silence for several hours. Every hour or so Don would poke his head in and grab the laptops that were ready and write the names of agents on them.

For the next two days, Mark and I worked together, sunup to sundown, to provide laptops to three squads—more than one hundred agents. And then . . .

"We have breaking news. Anthrax has been found in the post office on the Upper West Side." We all turned to the television Don had brought in and stopped to watch the news report. Our desk phones started ringing.

"All the agents are on their way to the hospital as a precaution," Ben said from across the room. He got up and rushed out of the office.

One of our squads had set up operations inside the post office. Thankfully they isolated the Anthrax to another floor, and the ventilation system was turned off at the time. The building was sealed off, however, along with all the squad's property.

Don hung up his phone and turned to Mark. "How many laptops do we have left?"

"Enough to cover them," Mark responded.

"Great. They'll be here in a few hours. Here are all the names. You and Sam take care of assigning them."

Mark tugged the back of my shirt, and we disappeared into the far office.

"Hey, guys." Don said, interrupting us. "You're doing a great job."

This never seems to end, I thought. *It's bad enough I have to drive past the freezer trucks every day, and now an Anthrax attack.*

Mark and I worked diligently to make sure the laptops were loaded with the correct software. We wrote the agents' names on sticky notes and placed each laptop, one after the other, on the tables which ran the length of the office.

"Yo, Sam." I heard someone yell my name from the other room.

"I'm in with the laptops," I responded.

Patrick came to the door. "Your new G-Ride is ready to go. You've been assigned to the JTTF for the next week. I need you to sign these papers."

I signed for my G-Ride, a silver Crown Victoria. *Nice*, I thought. Wilson was free from picking me up each morning, and I was off to my next assignment.

∽

I heard raised voices as soon as I opened the front door.

"What the fuck is your problem?"

"I don't have a problem, bud. You're the one with the problem. We're supposed to share this information."

I followed signs for the JTTF and discovered that I was the only female in a large conference room.

"Excuse me, gentlemen," I said as I walked into the room.

"Sorry, ma'am. Just a friendly disagreement."

"Don't mind me. I'm reporting as requested."

I took my seat at the table where the United States Secret Service placard identified my spot.

A casually dressed officer approached me. "Hi, I'm Maurice, NYPD."

"Hey, Maurice. I'm Sam, Secret Service. What's with those guys?" I asked, pointing to the door with my head.

"Oh, yeah, those guys. The big guy's my lieu [lieutenant], and the guy in the suit is FBI." Maurice explained that the FBI brought in their own trailer and were running telephone lines in there. "They disappear for hours on end, and my lieu found out they are not sharing any information. You guys are working the money angle, right?" he asked.

"Yeah. Does anyone else know about what the FBI is doing?" I asked.

"We just found out, so I'm not sure. You better inform your folks. Since you're a Fed too, your guys may get further than us."

"Understood," I said.

I stepped out of the JTTF Command Post and called Don. I filled him in on what Maurice told me and confirmed that there was no agent at the table with us.

"Motherfuckers!" he yelled.

I held the phone away from my ear as he continued to yell expletives.

"Let me get Ben on it. The SAIC may come down, so be on your toes, young lady, and get as much info as possible."

"I'm on it."

BACK TO WORK

Over the next few hours, I spoke to everyone around the table involved in the JTTF. They were happy to talk about the week's BS with the FBI and showed me where the wires were running.

"What did your boss say, Sam?" Maurice asked.

"My SAIC may come down," I said.

"He a big guy?"

"Sorry, Maurice, I'm not understanding. What do you mean?"

"Sometimes it takes a little physical intimidation—wink, wink," he said.

"Gotcha, Maurice. How about a 6'5" tall black guy who played college football?" All the guys looked up from the table.

"That'll do, Sam, that'll do." We high-fived.

The next day I reported straight to La Guardia and took my seat at the conference table for JTTF duty. Every now and then the phone rang, and I took information pertaining to the Anthrax attack at the Post Office. The guys and I spent the rest of the time sharing work stories. I was on the phone when my SAIC arrived. I didn't see him walk outside to the trailer.

"This is not how it works! You guys pack your stuff and get that trailer out of here now! Oh, and here's a letter from Giuliani's office. You can leave on your own, or the NYPD can help you leave—your choice."

There were some additional choice words exchanged on both sides, but that was the last time any of us saw the FBI at La Guardia.

"Agent Perper, a moment, please," my SAIC said.

I got up from my chair and met him outside the conference room door.

"Let's walk and talk," he suggested. He did most of the talking, and I listened.

He explained that the FBI had been asked to vacate this particular JTTF office and I was to take the call if someone asked to speak to the FBI agent in charge.

"Everyone else here is a team player. It looks like you all are collecting some good intel. Keep it up, Perper."

"Yes, sir, I will. Thank you."

He extended his giant football hand, and I shook it. You could barely see me when he stood in front of me and my hand disappeared in his grip.

"See you in the office next week," he said, as he turned and walked out the door.

I returned to the conference room. Maurice and the other guys were waiting for me.

"Sam, your SAIC *is* huge! Glad he was able to take care of business," said Maurice.

"Me, too," I responded. "I'm relieved that it went as smoothly as it did. You never know."

"True. Some guys just get on an ego trip and it's a mess."

I looked down at my watch. "Lunch, anyone?" I said.

"Sam, if it wasn't for you, I think I'd starve," said one of the officers.

"Yeah, I'm glad you don't eat salad!" Maurice chimed in. "The last group was mostly girls . . . no offense . . . and day after day, it was salad, salad, salad."

"No offense taken. Pizza, subs, deli?" I asked.

"Yes, please!" a voice said from across the room. We all laughed.

I picked up the phone and called Joey's Place, a popular spot with the NYPD. The JTTF picked up the tab while we were on duty.

BACK TO WORK

Thirty minutes later lunch arrived, and for the rest of the day we answered phones and each other's questions about our law enforcement lives. The week went by quickly. I looked forward to a Sunday off before returning to the office on Monday.

Working the JTTF allowed for more regular hours. I was home by seven in the evening, and the wine and beer flowed until bedtime. It was the only way I could sleep at this point without having nightmares or dreams of any kind. I didn't care what anyone said about it. In fact most of the agents were existing this way. In order for us to focus on the task at hand, we had to medicate our way through the nights—the exception being those assigned to nighttime duty.

I was really struggling with the commute into the city. The smells, the sounds, the freezer trucks all were a constant reminder of the hell I went through. I put my name in for out-of-town assignments and was fortunate to receive several two-week stints at the Clinton's residence in Chappaqua, New York.

Most of the assignments had me working midnights. At first it was difficult to adjust to nights—mostly because humans were meant to sleep at night and be awake during the day. A few days into an assignment, though, and I was able to reverse my sleep patterns. Additionally the hotel I stayed in was very quiet during the day, so I was able to fall asleep and stay asleep.

The Clinton's schedule dictated how busy I was at the residence. I would assist in prepping the house for arrivals and then make sure the house and property were secure after departures. The best part was that it was a more casual assignment in terms of dress code. Most of the time we dressed down in business casual, and when it got cold, we wore multiple layers, hats, gloves, and boots.

On occasion the Clinton's dog Buddy would come out of the house with a tennis ball, wanting to play. He had fetch down to a science, and he was smart. One particular day he intentionally knocked the tennis ball under one of the trucks in the motorcade and stood in front of it so we couldn't leave. One of the agents took his extendable baton and went under the truck. He came out with the ball and threw it as far as he could so we could leave before Buddy came back.

All in all these were not bad assignments, and I was thankful they got me out of the city where I felt like I could breathe a little easier.

PART TWO
FROM TRAUMA TO TRIUMPH

SEVEN

A ROCKY START

I TALKED TO Steve every evening. Our relationship was growing stronger, and as a result I wanted to be with him more and more. I couldn't wait to get home for the Thanksgiving holiday. My leave had been approved, and my personal vehicle was packed and ready to go. Wednesday at 5:00 p.m. rolled around, and I was off. Seven hours later I arrived at my mom's house in Maryland. After hugging her, I went right to the fridge for a beer. I had made sure to leave a stash behind after my last visit.

"What an insane drive back! There are too many people that live along the I-95 corridor."

"Oh, honey, I'm just glad you're home," my mom responded as she gave me a second hug.

It was midnight, and I was beat. After being trapped in a car for seven hours, I was in no mood to sit or sleep. I began feeling that familiar buzzing throughout my body, and I had to move. I grabbed another beer and walked over to Solomon who was asleep in his bed. I bent down and whispered in his ear.

"Come on, Soli. Let's go for a walk."

As soon as he heard the "W" word, he sprang out of his bed and ran to the top of the steps. I picked him up, put on his leash, and we ventured out into the cool, crisp November air. As we walked I took in the quiet and the scenery. The leaves in the trees had started to fall to the ground. The quiet was what I craved. Things continued to be very noisy in my world, and I wanted to stop that noise any way I could.

I returned to my mom's house, gave her another hug, and went into the kitchen for a third beer. I then went off to my room to get ready for bed. Solomon scampered behind me and scooted through the door before I closed it behind me. I put him up on the bed, turned on the television, and crawled under the covers with him. As the alcohol took effect, I feel asleep.

I woke mid-morning to the smell of sweet potatoes. It was Thanksgiving Day 2001, and I was looking forward to our family dinner. I made my way into the kitchen and started my coffee ritual.

"Good morning, sweetie," my mom said.

"Morning. Thanks for putting on the coffee, Mom."

I poured a cup, took a sip, and then gave my mom a big hug. "Everything smells so good!"

"Here, look." She turned on the oven light where I could see the potatoes cooking.

"Can I do the marshmallows?" I asked.

"Absolutely."

Each Thanksgiving my mom garnished her sweet potatoes with marshmallows, and either my sister or I put the marshmallows on top. My sister was not with us, so I won by default.

I inhaled the sweet, dark, golden yumminess that bubbled in the oven. I felt so good at this moment—the way things were when I was little, without a care in the world. I sipped my coffee, pulled up a small step stool, and sat in front of the oven. I waited,

A ROCKY START

I inhaled, I smelled the aroma, and I felt great. Solomon joined me in the kitchen. The peaceful atmosphere was complete.

A few hours later Steve and the rest of the family arrived. Nothing could spoil the way I felt.

With the table set and my marshmallows a golden brown, we sat down together and enjoyed Thanksgiving dinner. The conversation soon centered around me and my work. My peaceful atmosphere was slowly being eroded.

I excused myself, went to the kitchen, and brought back a bottle of wine. I poured glass after glass, numbing myself as the barrage of questions continued. It was not my family's fault—they were doing what any inquisitive family would do. They had not been with me in New York on 9/11, and they wanted to know the details. But after an hour of questions and almost a bottle of wine drunk, I excused myself and went to the bathroom.

I tried to think of a way to redirect this Thanksgiving dinner—to save it, to remember it as something I enjoyed as a child. I stayed in the bathroom a few extra minutes. Suddenly I noticed a trembling sensation. *Was a truck driving by the house?* I thought.

I put my hands on my quadriceps. *Oh, God, it's me!*

I looked in the mirror. I recognized my eyes, but it was as if I was looking into something hollow. I looked down at my hands. They weren't trembling. I looked at my arms. They weren't trembling either. *What the hell is going on?*

I could still feel the trembling, but nothing on the outside of my body matched what I was feeling on the inside. "Get it together, Sam," I told myself firmly.

I turned on the sink and splashed water on my face. "C'mon, girl. You got this."

While I was in training, I used to talk to myself before an exam, whether written or physical. I found it helped me to "get centered" and focus on the task at hand. I took a few deep breaths and concentrated on the aromas that filled the house. I took myself back to when I was a kid and the things I loved most about Thanksgiving. Those wonderful marshmallows! I smiled and opened my eyes. The trembling seemed to dissipate. I left the bathroom and returned to the table. Steve put his arm around me.

"Everything okay?" he asked.

"Yeah, I'm good," I replied, smiling. "Could you please pass the sweet potatoes?"

After everyone said their good-byes, Steve stayed to help me and my mom clean up. As I was washing some dishes, he came up behind me and wrapped his arms around my waist. He whispered in my ear, "How are you doing?"

"I'm great!" I replied enthusiastically. "It was fun being with everyone." By this time, between the alcohol and the delicious food, I *was* feeling great—because I wasn't feeling anything at all. I sensed that Steve wanted to ask me something, but he kept quiet. After we finished cleaning up, I walked Steve to his car.

"Let's go to Brookside Gardens tomorrow," he said as we hugged good night.

Brookside Gardens was a favorite destination in the community. It had creative, beautiful gardens which changed with the seasons. In the fall when the leaves were turning, the gardens were decorated for Thanksgiving and then for Christmas. In the summer the gardens were left alone to bloom beautifully. You could picnic, run or walk on the trail, or find a special corner and just hang out and take it all in.

A ROCKY START

"That sounds good. I love you," I told Steve, kissing him.

"Love you, too," he said after the kiss.

I watched him pull out of the driveway and head down the street. When his taillights disappeared, I walked back inside my mom's house. The aroma of Thanksgiving dinner still hung in the air.

My mom was in the laundry room, pretreating stains on the tablecloths. "I'm going to watch some television and get ready for bed," I said with a yawn. I thanked her for the delicious dinner and let her know that tomorrow Steve and I were planning a quiet afternoon at Brookside Gardens followed by dinner so I wouldn't be home until late.

"Okay, you guys have fun," she said with a smile.

&

Steve proposed in November 2001, and I accepted. Our wedding took place the following January—nothing elaborate, just a small ceremony at Steve's house in Maryland surrounded by our family and closest friends, followed by a party at a quaint, historic French restaurant. It was not your typical wedding. I had to be back in New York, so our honeymoon would have to wait.

Five days after Steve and I were married, my grandfather, Papa Harry, died. He was the strong, silent glue that held our family together. He spoke only if there was something important to say, someone asked for counsel, or he was watching golf on television. He knew all the stats on each golfer. He taught me how to swing a golf club when I was five years old. While I never took up the game, I learned to have an appreciation for it.

His death was a huge blow to the family. What made it especially difficult for me was that he died of a heart attack. The survivor guilt I carried with me from 9/11 created a belief that if I had been there, I could have saved him. I had the skill set. I was well versed in triage, first aid, and field treatment.

The reality was that this was my grandfather's fourth heart attack. He never should have survived number three, and this time his heart just gave out. He collapsed on the floor in Nordstrom's while shopping with my grandmother. (The family joke is that my grandmother "shopped" him to death.) I felt the loss deeply. It added to the grief I was already trying to deal with on a daily basis. The constant news coverage coupled with the ongoing investigation made it virtually impossible for me to focus on anything.

After our wedding I returned to New York. It would be nine months before we were able to get away, and I would spend the next three months separated from my new husband.

Exhausted, and in need of a change, my supervisor provided me with the opportunity. The New York Field Office needed a handful of agents to work the 2002 Olympic Winter Games in Salt Lake City. It meant a month on the road, and I quickly volunteered after talking with Steve. He had been part of the medical staff for the 1996 Summer Games in Atlanta and raved about his experience. I could not wait to get on the plane.

That February was one of the highlights of my career. The collaborative effort between the law enforcement agencies from around the United States, the United States military, and the public produced the most secure Olympic Games on record. It also was a breath of fresh air, literally. The scenery was spectacular; the athletes were a joy to be around. I felt hopeful again. We were outfitted head to toe to help combat the very cold temperatures—especially at night when it averaged ten to fifteen degrees below zero. That outerwear remains in my closet today as a reminder of one of the best experiences of my life.

Upon my return to New York, I felt renewed. The feeling did not last long.

While I was away, I made a decision to put in for a transfer to the Washington, DC, Field Office. Since Steve was a doctor and licensed to practice in Maryland, Virginia, and DC, it was only logical that I relocate. After several weeks of waiting, I discovered that logic and the United States Secret Service did not go together. My transfer was denied because, as the Service deemed, I had not put enough time in at the New York Field Office—this despite the need for agents in Washington, DC.

Could something just work out for a change so I can get on with my life? I thought.

I felt trapped. It seemed that no matter what I did to try and improve my mental state, I was met with a brick wall. I continued to put in for out of town and travel assignments. My habit of drinking to cope also continued, and I became more and more withdrawn. I went to work, did my time in the city each day, and then drove home. I declined any after-work activities with my squad mates, afraid that we would all be too drunk to make it home. When I got home, my routine was to make dinner or work out, plop in front of the TV with a bottle of something, wait until it took effect, and then head to bed.

I existed this way for months, cutting down on my drinking only if I was on assignment. The next big assignment came in March 2002: traveling internationally with President Bush. I took a military transport flight south into Mexico where President and First Lady Laura Bush, Vice President and Mrs. Cheney, and Secretary of State Condoleeza Rice were meeting with then-President Vincente Fox and his cabinet.

I was excited because it was my first international trip and it allowed me to get out of New York. Monterrey, Mexico, was beautiful. The architecture was captivating, and I found myself wandering around town on my off-time, taking in the sights and sounds. The travel bug had bitten me. I figured that, once back to New York, I would keep on top of all travel assignments and put my name in as soon as they were posted. Fortunately, the president's ranch in Crawford, Texas, posted frequently.

Eight agents from different field offices and I gathered together and boarded the white vans waiting for us outside Dallas/Fort Worth International Airport. With the air-conditioning blasting, we made our way to the Dallas Field Office for our briefing before heading down to the ranch.

"Hey, ya'll! Go on in there," a short, blonde-haired woman at the front desk said, pointing to the conference room.

That's quite the accent, I thought. I hadn't heard anyone say "ya'll" since I visited family in Savannah, Georgia, many years ago.

During the briefing we were all surprised to find out that we could wear shorts if we wanted as long as we had our duty boots to protect us from the snakes. Snakes? It was the first time I was on an assignment where we were briefed on wildlife, insects, and varmints we might encounter.

I looked around at my fellow agents. They all had similar puzzled looks. "Are we still in the U.S., or are we going into the Amazon?" one agent remarked.

Everyone laughed. "Ya'll will see what I'm talkin' about when you get out there," the senior agent said. "You got some drivin' to do, so you best be on ya'll's way."

We got up from the conference table and walked back toward the front office door.

"Oh, and watch out for the tarantulas!" the senior agent yelled. We stopped in our tracks.

"Did he say *tarantula*?" I muttered to the group. I stood at the door, trying to process the idea of coming face to face with a big, hairy spider. *Snakes and spiders. What kind of assignment did I volunteer for?* I thought to myself.

We pulled into our hotel a few hours later and walked across to the convenience store. With a decent-sized fridge in the room, I could stock up on alcohol for the week. I was surprised that every agent I was with purchased at least a six-pack. The job took its toll on all of us, it seemed. I retired to my room, popped a frozen dinner into the microwave, and guzzled my first beer, finishing it before my dinner was done cooking.

"Ah, that is perfect," I said to myself as I looked at the beer bottle. I turned on the television, grabbed another beer, and ate my dinner. Before long the six-pack was gone, and I was ready to sleep. I continued this same routine for the rest of the week while I was in Texas.

I returned to New York to find my office in a flurry of activity. A raid was planned for the evening, and it was all hands on deck. Before I could say hello, a new ballistic vest landed in my arms.

"Shotgun or sidearm?" my supervisor asked.

"Sidearm," I responded.

"Mark, you got the shotgun!" my supervisor yelled to the agent in the other room.

We were headed to Queens to serve a warrant for fraud involving bogus telephone cards. Real numbers had been stolen, and the perp created and sold telephone calling cards, passing them off as genuine.

I got home at 2:00 a.m., completely exhausted. Too tired to make dinner, I drank a few beers and fell into bed. The alarm clock awakened me a few hours later. After silencing it I rolled over and thought, *There's got to be more than this in life.*

I had worked so hard to become an agent. But now nothing about the job was rewarding anymore. I felt like a dark cloud was following me all the time. If I was not at work, I was drinking so I would be able to go to work. While I was at work, I couldn't concentrate. I would sit in front of my computer and stare at the reports. I longed to get a weekend off so I could visit Steve. Every attempt to secure a day off was met by another in-town assignment.

Later that day I picked up the phone and called Beverly, the Human Resources counselor.

"Hello, is this Beverly?" I said softly as I cupped the lower part of the phone so no one could overhear. When she said yes, I told her I needed to speak with her. I explained it all—the drinking, the nightmares, the constant stress, my failed attempt at a transfer, and how I felt about my job.

She said that she and several others in her office were planning a return trip to New York to "check in" with those who wanted to meet, but it was several months out.

"Keep my number, Samantha. Call me anytime. Hang in there," she said.

A ROCKY START

I hung up the phone. *Hang in there?* I thought. Stellar words of advice to a person who was barely able to function.

Feeling completely unsupported and deflated, I left the office, drove to the liquor store, and then went home and drank my way to sleep.

※

Two weeks later I finally got a weekend off, and Steve decided to come to New York, saving me the drive. He asked if I could take him and his parents down to Ground Zero, and I agreed. Steve and I met his parents at a designated time at the corner of Church and Vesey Streets. The entire area was fenced off, and I made my way to the NYPD officer standing at the gate. I introduced myself and asked if he could let me through with three others. At first he declined. I told him I completely understood and then mentioned that I had worked in 7 World Trade, which was now a rubble heap. He got his lieutenant, and they ushered us in. The lieutenant told us to watch our footing, and told me that I was responsible for my guests. I thanked him again and shook his hand.

The four of us walked down Vesey Street in silence. Steve's parents held hands as they walked. Steve and I walked separately so I could point out where buildings used to be and any hazards we needed to watch out for.

The fires continued to burn. We walked as far down Vesey Street as we could and stopped in front of where 7 WTC used to be. There were papers all over the place. Several FDNY firefighters were sifting through a pile of rubble. They stopped when they saw us approach.

"Hey, officer," one of the firefighters said to me.

THE SILENT FALL

"Hey. What's up?" I responded as I shook his hand.

"You guys will need these if you're gonna be down here," he said, handing us masks to cover our noses and mouths.

"Thanks," I said as I passed them to Steve and his parents.

The firefighter and I started a conversation. I told him I had worked in 7 WTC. He mentioned that he and his crew had been battling with putting the fire out in that building, and that it sounded like random gunshots were being fired. I told him what was inside the building—guns, ammunition, and other things that could "cook off" or create small explosions. It was certainly reasonable that the heat from the fires caused the ammunition to charge and go off.

"Well, that explains a lot. Thank you, ma'am."

"No problem. Sir, can I ask you a question?" I said, removing my mask. "Could the heat from the jet fuel make the towers collapse?"

He paused for a moment and then explained that the amount of jet fuel that continued to pour into the buildings created a fire that burned so hot that it destabilized the structures significantly—enough that they could not continue to remain intact.

"Every time we move a large amount of debris, the fires reignite. It's bad," he said.

We looked at the massive amount of debris in front of us. Some was so high it was like looking at small mountains. Every time I came across papers containing personal information, I thought about the person. *Is he or she somewhere in this pile?*

I looked down and saw a chunk of what used to be the floor of 7 WTC. I picked it up and brushed it off.

"Hey, sir! Is it okay if I keep this?" I asked, holding up the piece of the floor.

A ROCKY START

"You bet," he responded, giving me a thumbs-up.

It was incredibly loud with all the machinery running. As we walked further down Vesey Street, we realized we were running out of space to navigate. A police lieutenant stopped us and informed us that we could not proceed any farther because of the fire burning ahead. He let us out of the gate and directed us toward the Red Cross tents which were set up on the West Side Highway.

The Red Cross tent city was manned 24/7. It was a mobile command post for the rescue and recovery efforts, and it provided rescue workers with a place to eat, sleep, and clean up after their shifts. All visitors and volunteers were required to check in before walking into Ground Zero and check out when departing.

Steve and I walked his parents back to their car and said our good-byes. They thanked me for taking the personal time with them.

Steve and I walked a few blocks in silence.

"Sam, I want to help. These guys need support for what they are doing," Steve said, breaking the silence between us.

I suggested that he bring his portable chiropractic table down and give adjustments to the rescue personnel and any members of the NYPD or FDNY. Steve liked the idea.

The next morning we got up and went back to Ground Zero, chiropractic table in tow. We checked in at the Red Cross tent. Steve grabbed one of the team leaders and mentioned that he would like to offer his services. The team leader gave him a place to set up, and Steve went to work. I was offered a mask because the air was filled with smoke and dust, but I declined. I watched as Steve offered relief to the folks that took him up on his offer to help.

One of the officers with the NYPD saw my raid jacket and invited me into the mess tent for coffee. The raid jackets were provided by headquarters, and each of us had received one. Adorned with the lettering "United States Secret Service and Police" in bright yellow, the black jackets clearly identified us.

"So is that guy your husband?" the officer asked as he handed me a cup of coffee.

I smiled. "Yeah. We got married in January."

"That's great. How long has he been a chiro?" he asked.

"Almost twenty years." *I am being interviewed before this guy lets Steve adjust him,* I thought.

"He any good?" the officer asked.

"I married him, didn't I?" I said, laughing. "Seriously though, he's the best. He keeps me in one piece. You know how it is—the body armor and all the equipment. I'd be a mess without regular adjustments. Let him work on you. I promise you'll feel better."

"I think I will," the officer said as he downed his coffee.

"C'mon, I'll introduce you. I'm Sam, by the way," I said, extending my hand.

"Glad to meet you, Sam. I'm Gino."

I introduced Gino to Steve and let Steve go to work on him. I returned to the mess tent for more coffee. While pouring a fresh cup, another NYPD officer introduced himself to me. He knew several agents I worked with, and we struck up a conversation. While Steve continued to work on Gino, the officer and I walked down to Ground Zero.

A few hours later Steve and I were both beat and very hungry. We declined the offer to eat in the mess tent; we didn't dare consume the rescuers' valuable commodities.

A ROCKY START

As we were walking out, Gino stopped me. "You guys taking off?"

"Yeah, we're going to grab some food up the street and then head back to Jersey," I said.

"You've got to go to my friend's place up the street. Best food in the city. Chambers and West Broadway."

"Sounds perfect. Great meeting you, Gino. Stay safe."

"You too, Sam. Thanks a bunch, Doc!" He said, waving goodbye.

We entered the small restaurant. I was a bit embarrassed because of the way I was dressed. I stuck out in my raid jacket, duty boots, black tactical pants, and my baseball cap. The host did not seem to notice and sat us at a corner table.

The waiter came over and introduced himself. He placed water and fresh baked bread on the table. We ordered based on the waiter's recommendations and received our food quickly.

"Gino was right," I said to Steve. It was some of the best food I had ever eaten in the city.

The waiter came over and asked if we wanted anything else. "Please tell the chef that the food was outstanding," I said.

The waiter said he would, and a few minutes later, the chef appeared at our table. "I want to thank you for coming in and for your service, ma'am. Please enjoy this dessert on the house."

"Thank you so much; that is so sweet of you. This meal was a bright spot amidst all of this chaos, and I appreciate that you are open and serving the community. It means a lot that you would come down here every day."

I could tell I had struck a nerve. Blushing, he looked down

at the floor. When he looked up he had tears in his eyes, which immediately made me tear up. Steve followed right behind.

"I lost a lot of friends with both departments. It is in their honor that I keep my doors open—a way to say thank you."

"You honor us all, sir. Thank you," I said. We stood and shook each other's hands. When we walked out the door, I sat down on the curb and cried. Steve sat down next to me and put his arm around me.

We walked together for a while after that and returned to my apartment several hours later. Steve was going back to Maryland in the morning, and I wanted him to get a good night's rest after such an emotional day. We did not talk much about what we had seen and experienced, choosing to hold each other and enjoy the quiet.

The next morning Steve left. My heart was heavy; I did not know when I would see him again.

EIGHT

REALITY CHECK

IT WAS THE beginning of another workweek, and I was elated to discover that I would have some time off the following week and could go home to Maryland.

I started my drive at 2:00 a.m. Saturday morning, having just ended a protective assignment with Vice President and Mrs. Cheney in New York.

At 5:00 a.m. I pulled in Steve's driveway and quietly snuggled into bed with him. It felt so good to come home to him. At noon I woke up and stumbled into the bathroom. I splashed some water on my face and was startled by my appearance in the mirror. The dark circles under my eyes revealed the utter exhaustion I felt.

I made my way to the kitchen where Steve was eating lunch. "Hey there, sleepyhead. I didn't dare wake you," he said. Gratefully I let him wrap his arms around me. We stood in the middle of the kitchen and swayed back and forth.

"Coffee," I said, breaking the embrace.

"Right there. I turned in on not twenty minutes ago, so it's still fairly fresh."

I grabbed the biggest mug Steve had in his cupboard, filled it to the brim, and quickly drank almost half of it before sitting at the table. Steve brought his lunch over and sat down next to me. "I'm glad you're here," he said.

"Me, too," I responded with a smile.

"You look really tired, Sam."

"I am. Things are just so crazy at work. I can't seem to catch a break. I'm glad to be here now."

For whatever reason I did not say anything to Steve about the chaos that continued both at work and inside me. I made the choice to hide my downward spiral from the closest people in my life, determined to get through this myself, the way I had always done. I believed the ridiculously flawed logic I had heard growing up: "If you don't talk about it, it (whatever it is) will never happen."

I had spent so much of my life "sucking it up" and putting my best face forward that I did not know any other way to be. My well had run dry. I was out of energy to keep "sucking it up." Inside my head swirled thoughts about giving up, giving in, and running away. But I couldn't; it went against who I was. *Sam does not give up. Sam puts her head down and drives forward with a force to be reckoned with.* At times my force left friends and family so alienated, it would be years before we could speak again.

I relied on my medication—alcohol—to numb me to the thoughts and voices that wanted to defeat me. What I did not realize was that the amount of alcohol I was consuming was poisoning me inside and out. At this point I was a master at keeping it hidden, though. I never went to work drunk or with a hangover. I did not drink excessively around family and friends, and I was never drunk in public.

The weekend with Steve went by quickly. We spent the time relaxing together, watching movies, and cuddling on the couch.

REALITY CHECK

I arrived at my apartment in New Jersey late Sunday evening and prepared for work the following morning. I fell sleep easily after drinking a half a bottle of red wine. At 3:00 a.m. I woke up. Lying awake in bed, I stared at the ceiling. *What the hell am I going to do?* I wondered.

The images of the terrorists pinned to the whiteboard in my office came one after the other. It was always Mohammad Atta that got my blood to boil. Now fully awake, I got out of bed, showered, dressed, and headed to the office. I arrived at 4:30 a.m. Surprisingly I found my supervisor and several agents working away.

"Hey, Sam. What are you doing here so early?" Don asked.

"Hey, Don. Couldn't sleep, so I thought I'd get some work done."

"Me neither. You okay?" he said.

"Yeah," I replied, lying through my teeth. I was pretty sure that everyone in the office was experiencing the same things I was, but no one mentioned it. It was ultimately the silence, the lack of talking about it that led to the spiraling, silent fall from being at the top of my game. Eventually seven other agents would join me in leaving the New York Field Office.

By spring 2002 I had had enough. I was glued to the field office, unable to get any travel assignments. Beverly's visit to "check in" on us was unremarkable and not helpful. I was completely depleted and numb to everything all the time. I didn't care about anything or anyone. I saw the Secret Service as a cold, calculated enemy that couldn't care less about the health and well-being of its agents who dedicated their lives to "the job."

I sat down at my computer and drafted my resignation. I placed it in an interoffice envelope and waited for the ATSAIC to contact me. Two weeks later I was in his office turning in my issued equipment.

"Are you sure you want to do this, Sam? We spent a lot of money training you," he said.

Shocked, I looked him straight in the eye. "With all due respect, sir, my decision is far removed from money. But you could keep me on if you simply granted my transfer to DC."

I was absolutely appalled that someone I considered a friend would make this about money. It was clear that those in charge of the New York Field Office were unable to comprehend—or simply chose not to see—what was happening to the agents around them.

"I'm sorry, Sam, that's out of my hands," he said.

"Then we really do not have anything else to talk about."

I took out my credentials and looked at them for the last time. I thought about how hard I had worked to earn them. I closed my eyes, took a deep breath, and placed them facedown on the table along with my duty weapon. I turned in the keys to my G-ride, signed the property log, and walked out.

My squad mate, Wilson, was waiting in the lobby to drive me home. "You okay, Sam?" he asked.

"I don't know right this second. Let's go," I responded.

We sat in silence for most of the drive home. He asked me what our ATSAIC said. When I told him, he too was surprised he tried to make it about money.

We pulled into the parking lot of my building. "I want to thank you, Wilson, for everything, for being my friend. I'll miss you. I wish you all the best in your career," I said, extending my hand.

Wilson took it and replied, "I'll miss you, too, Sam. Be well in your journey. I wish you and Steve a happy marriage together."

I got out of the car and watched Wilson pull away for the last time.

I walked up to my apartment and picked up the phone. "Hey, Steve. What are you doing for the rest of your life?"

Steve laughed on the other end.

"I'm coming home," I said.

I arranged for a one-way U-Haul, and within two weeks I had everything packed. I paid my landlord for breaking the lease, even though he did not require it, and my career as a United States Secret Service Agent assigned to the New York Field Office officially ended. Four and a half hours later, I was unpacking at Steve's home in Maryland.

I avoided friends and my extended family until I was completely settled. Steve went to work each day, and I tended to the house. It was a big adjustment for both of us. It was wonderful to finally be with my husband, but still uncomfortable enough that I had to call him at his office to ask if I could move his stuff to make room for mine.

Although I had changed locations, my drinking continued as a way to cope with the adjustment to civilian life. The adjustment was made more difficult because it was the beginning of the thunderstorm season. At the first sound of thunder or flash of lightning, my heart would race. I often found myself crouched on the floor or in a corner with Steve's arms around me. I could not drink this fear away. It sent my mind spinning. I had no control and I hated it. On one particular summer evening, a severe storm blew right over the house. Both Steve and I were in the kitchen next to the sliding glass doors which led to the elevated deck.

BOOM!

I jumped back in fear and cowered in the corner. Steve rushed over to me.

"You're safe, Sam. I've got you," he said.

"Just make it stop. Please make it stop," I cried.

I could not move; I was paralyzed. Steve covered me, keeping himself between me and the glass door until the storm passed. It felt like an eternity. He did not leave my side the reminder of the evening.

After that storm I became homebound. I went outside only to walk my dog Solomon and only if there was zero threat of a storm. I thought that leaving the Secret Service was the most difficult decision I had made in my life, but I was not prepared for what lay ahead.

༺༻

The summer of 2002 was bittersweet. Here I was, free to do and pursue anything I wanted, and all I could do was sleep. I averaged twelve hours of sleep for one solid month. If I was not sleeping, I was in front of the television drinking. If there was a thunderstorm, Steve was by my side doing his best to distract me. Occasionally we would go out to dinner, but only if the weather was clear. Each bill Steve paid showed a bar tab at least twice the price of the meal with drinks flowing before, during, and after. We would get home, and I would grab a nightcap before retiring to bed.

Steve was not prepared for the woman he married to live like this. "Sam, are you sure you're okay?" he asked a million times. Every time my answer was the same. "Yeah, I just need to take the edge off." I literally felt as though I was clinging to the edge of a cliff. My fingers were slipping, and I was barely hanging on. Every day I would wake up and promise myself that I would be a better wife. That I was going to lay off the booze. Every day I broke those promises.

A small sliver of happiness came in October, when Steve and I finally went on our honeymoon. We chose Ambergris Caye, an island off the coast of Belize, after a friend recommended it. It was spectacular. The island was alive—the air, the water, the food, the vegetation, the animals. Every day was a new adventure. I chose to be present to these new adventures by not consuming alcohol until evening. Drinking was still the only way I knew to stop the nightmares.

When it was time to return home, I was completely bummed. I thought about what it would be like to relocate to Belize, and I mentioned it to Steve. Island life seemed simpler. No car needed. Shoes were optional everywhere, and as countries go Belize had a stable government and currency.

Steve was surprised that I would even consider moving to a different country. After doing some research when we returned home, we decided to keep visiting but put any plans to relocate on hold. The decision was a good one. Hurricane season of 2003 was tough for Belize; the island took a beating.

The last few weeks of 2002 were miserable. It had been cold and rainy for a number of days. I had hit bottom. I was ready to let go of the cliff. I had lost myself; I felt completely hopeless. All

I could see was a failed career, the death of my grandfather, and my PTSD, which was out of control. I shut everything out. I felt like no one understood. I was angry. I felt trapped in a world that was alien to me. Nothing made sense anymore. At night, in the darkness, I'd cry myself to sleep, wondering if I'd ever be happy again. "What's the point?" I asked myself over and over again.

After ushering in 2003 with a few friends at the house, I kissed Steve good night and went downstairs. I had drunk enough to take the edge off, but not enough to numb myself. I took two bottles of wine and a glass downstairs to the basement and turned on the TV. As I drank I watched everyone on TV celebrate the New Year. *If I have to live another year like this, I won't survive*, I thought.

Through my alcohol-induced haze, I thought about how life would be without the pain and the daily frustrations. I thought about life without me in it. I so craved peace, and I wondered if the only way I could achieve it was to end my time here on earth. I had hidden my fall to the bottom from everyone except Steve and my mom.

"They won't miss me. They can go on without me. It's not like I'm around anyway," I said to myself. I picked up my gun and put it to my head. I closed my eyes and slipped my finger onto the trigger. I burst into tears and put the gun down. I poured another glass of wine and gulped it down in the hopes it would give me courage to pull the trigger. I picked up my gun again and put the barrel against my right temple. "Please, I just want it to stop," I cried out, and I started to squeeze the trigger.

I heard a voice say, "It's not your time. Sam, it's not your time."

REALITY CHECK

With tears streaming down my face, I dropped the gun on my lap. "God, please help me," I said in response to the voice.

Solomon came down the steps and walked over to me. He looked up at me and then down at the gun in my lap. I put the gun aside and scooped him up into my lap. I held him and cried until I passed out.

A few hours later I woke up. I sat up, not recognizing my surroundings. My gun and two empty wine bottles lay on the floor next to me. Solomon was still at my side, asleep. He opened his eyes when I tried to move. I pulled myself off the floor and walked into the bathroom, where I splashed water on my face. I put the empty bottles in the recycling bin and put my gun back in its case. I picked Solomon up and carried him upstairs. I quietly crawled under the covers, making sure I did not wake Steve.

When I opened my eyes again and looked at the clock, it was two in the afternoon. Solomon was in bed with me. My head was pounding. I wrapped myself in my bathrobe and wandered groggily downstairs to the kitchen. Coffee was first on the agenda.

Steve was in the basement with my mom. He came upstairs when he heard me in the kitchen. I was savoring my cup of coffee with both hands wrapped around the mug. He leaned over me from behind, wrapped his arms around me, and gave me a kiss on the cheek.

"Happy New Year, Sam. I love you," he whispered.

"I love you, too," I said, putting my mug down. I stood up and hugged him. I put my head on his shoulder, and we stayed there until we were interrupted by my mom.

"Sorry, you two. I wanted to wish my baby a Happy New Year," she said.

I went from hugging Steve to hugging my mom. "Thanks, Mom. Love you."

I spent the rest of the day watching movies, cuddled up on the couch with Solomon. I never mentioned my suicide attempt. I continued to push everything further down into the empty hole of my soul, determined to figure it out on my own and ashamed that I had allowed things get this bad. I could not help thinking about the voice that told me it was not my time. What was I supposed to do now?

Winter turned to spring, and spring to summer. All the promises I made to do better went unfulfilled, with the exception of getting back to an exercise routine. Physical exercise provided my brain with the endorphins it so desperately lacked. Those energetic endorphins allowed me to better get through the day and not feel the need to drink as much.

Nights continued to be met with the fear of nightmares. I stopped going to bed when Steve did, choosing to drink until I felt that I had completely shut my brain down. I was up to two bottles of wine a night. By the end of each week, our recycling bin looked as though Steve and I had thrown a party.

One summer morning I awoke to find Steve and my mom talking in the living room.

"Morning, Mom. This is a nice surprise," I said.

I exchanged hugs with both of them and went into the kitchen to grab some coffee. I came back to the living room and sat on the couch.

"Sam, we need to talk with you about something," Steve said.

"Okay, what's up?" I replied, curious to hear what was next.

"I could not help but notice the recycling bin and how much

you are drinking. I know it's been a rough time, but I feel like you're not even here anymore—it's like you've checked out."

I looked down at the floor. I could not even look at my own husband as he went on to describe how he felt like he'd lost the person he married.

Then my mom chimed in. "Honey, we want you to get some help. I know someone I think may be able to help."

I couldn't say anything except "okay." A surge of emotion flooded my body. My mom sat down next to me on the couch and reassured me that everything would be all right. She put a piece of paper with a name and a number written on it down on the coffee table.

"I love you," she said as she hugged me.

"I love you too, Mom," I managed to say.

She got up from the couch and walked out the front door. Steve sat down next to me and put his arm around me. I rested my head on his shoulder. We sat in silence.

"I'm sorry," I said, putting my hand on Steve's knee. "I didn't mean to shut you out. I've tried to fix this so many times. Can you forgive me?"

"Just get some help, Sam—please," he responded, pleading with me.

"Okay," I said, looking down at the floor. I had nothing to lose except my mind, such as it was. Which was a good thing.

NINE

NEW BEGINNINGS

"HI, SAM. COME on in," she said with a smile.

I walked into Harriet's office and looked around, immediately noticing some gadgets in the corner I was unfamiliar with. The space was nicely appointed and warm. The different shades of green went well with the dark wood furniture. Harriet invited me to sit down and elaborate on why I called and requested her services. She told me she was going to take notes and reassured me that everything I shared with her was confidential.

I started by taking her through the events of September 11, 2001. When I got to the part about the collapse of WTC Tower Two, there was a loud bang just outside her office. I jumped sky high. My body surged with adrenaline. I could feel my heart pounding so hard I thought it would jump out of my chest. I started to sweat.

I looked at Harriet. She was talking to me—I could see her lips moving, but I couldn't hear her. My eyes began to fill with tears. I couldn't move or speak; I just sat there, feeling helpless. Inside my head, my brain was screaming at me to speak, but I couldn't.

Harriet reached out and touched my knee. "Sam, Sam. Come back. You are safe here. It's okay. You are safe," she said.

I blinked, and the tears streamed down my face. I looked at her and shook my head no.

I could feel my body shaking. Harriet moved closer to me.

"Breathe," she said softly, keeping her hand on my knee.

I slowly returned to the present. "I'm sorry," I said.

"There's no need to apologize," she responded. "You are in my office, and you are in a safe place. Do you think you can continue?" she asked as she handed me some water.

"I think so," I responded. I proceeded to take her through the entire day. She asked about my reactions to things, similar to what she had just witnessed in her office. I told her about the thunderstorms, the nightmares, my reticence to leave my house, the drinking.

She handed me some more water and began to explain what Post Traumatic Stress Disorder was. She said I was displaying some of PTSD's classic symptoms: being hypervigilant—so alert to everything around me that my brain was on constant processing overload. She assured me that she could help me with a treatment protocol called EMDR (Eye Movement Desensitization Reprocessing), something that had worked successfully for Vietnam veterans. She would, in essence, reprogram my brain to function as it did prior to me experiencing the trauma.

"You mean I'd be able to be my old self again, like I was before 9/11?" I asked.

"That would be our goal, Sam," she responded.

"Then let's do this."

The treatment was unlike anything I had ever experienced. This was no "sit on the couch and tell me your problems"-type of therapy. I followed lights that would track back and forth with my eyes. The vibrating paddles I had in my hands would pulsate in a certain sequence as well. Stress responses were measured on a scale of one to ten.

I reported to Harriet's office two to three times a week. She had me relive 9/11 over and over again. For the first two weeks, I thought I would go crazy. I could not sleep, and I continued to drink heavily. I told Harriet I was not sure I could continue.

"Sam, you are the toughest person I know. Look what you went through to become an agent, what you put your body through. You can do this. I promise you this works, and it will get easier."

I trusted her and her track record. By the end of the first month, I was experiencing some relief; I started sleeping through the night and was consuming much less alcohol.

By the end of month three, although loud booming sounds still bothered me, I did not experience any flashbacks and wasn't reliving the events of 9/11. I was able, with Steve's help, to stay conscious and present to my surroundings.

Dealing with the anger and survivor's guilt was a deeper process. I was continuously frustrated with people who just "didn't get it." All the political bullshit and banter back and forth fed my anger. Those who were ignorant about the events of 9/11 made me seethe. Those who talked conspiracy made my blood boil. It was if they had forgotten that almost three thousand people had been murdered.

There was an undercurrent of stress that ran continuously through my body. Sometimes I could feel it and sometimes not. On one particular occasion, I was sitting on the couch in Harriet's office. We had just finished a session, and I asked her if the subway ran under her office because I felt like the floor was shaking. She said no and then she touched my knee. I was trembling. To the naked eye, my body didn't seem to be doing anything. On the inside I was a mess. Cortisol, the body's stress hormone, was on a rampage within me.

It took a few months to make a dent in my anger and frustration. Losing my grandfather in the midst of everything and the feelings surrounding that event surprisingly played a big part in my treatment. Harriet explained that not only did I have survivor's guilt over 9/11, but I also harbored it over the loss of my grandfather. I believed that if I was there when he collapsed that I could have saved him. She insisted that we make this part of my EMDR treatment as well.

The biggest breakthrough came when there was a thunderstorm and I did not feel like I had to dive for cover. I was hugely relieved and began leaving the house for extended periods of time. I started to feel like I was getting my life back.

As time went on my sleep-filled nights increased minus the nightmares, and the amount I was drinking significantly decreased.

I experienced a few bumps in the road along the way. One day there was a huge warehouse fire nearby. I happened to be driving with the windows open and could smell the sour stench of burning concrete. It was the same as the smell on 9/11 and for the months following as the fires burned. My heart began to pound and I started to sweat. I was taken back for a split second, but I willed my way back to the present. I pulled into a parking lot to slow my heart rate. All the "tricks" I learned in my EMDR treatment were working. I told Steve what happened.

NEW BEGINNINGS

"I'm proud of you, Sam," he said with a big smile.

"I'm proud of me, too," I responded.

And that day I did not feel the need to reach for a beer or a glass of wine to take the edge off. It was a memorable milestone.

As the months went on, I acquired more tools to manage my hypervigilance and stress responses. There were no more flashbacks or nightmares. I was startled by the same things everyone else was. By the summer of 2004 I had returned. EMDR literally saved my life. I will be forever grateful to Steve and my mom for their gentle intervention and to Harriet, who with care and compassion brought "the real me" back.

☙

I was eager to get back to work. Back into a career. Back to feeling like I made a difference. *If I keep myself immersed in something, I'll be okay,* I thought.

During the summer of 2002, Steve and I took a trip to Alpharetta, Georgia, to be trained on how to run our new sports performance franchise. I had found my calling—I was the owner and ran all the day-to-day operations. We were a standout in the community, offering a unique way for athletes to train. This was a true athletic performance center. It was 15,000 square feet of turf, track, top-of-the-line Eleiko weight plates, and four full-sized Power Systems racks. We offered a timing system utilizing the latest and greatest technology, and I had a full staff of highly qualified, hand-selected trainers. I was "on task" and in control.

And then I wasn't.

After returning home from a long day at the center, I woke up with a pounding headache and a loss of vision in my right eye. *Oh*

THE SILENT FALL

no, not again, I thought, remembering what had happened three years earlier.

Back in 1999 I woke up one morning and thought I had scratched my eye during the night. The bottom half of the vision in my right eye was affected. Several hours later I sat in my eye doctor's office expecting to receive some sort of prescription eyedrops.

"I don't like what I see," my doctor said, looking concerned. "I'm going to refer you to one of my colleagues."

"Okay. It's not serious, is it?" I asked.

"Your optic nerve is enlarged, and I want my colleague examine you. He's seen this before," she responded.

The next day I had an appointment with her colleague. I was convinced that I had some sort of infection that would probably require some antibiotics.

Two hours later a battery of tests confirmed I had optic neuritis, inflammation of the optic nerve. As a consequence, I had temporarily lost the bottom half of the vision in my right eye, and both my eye and head hurt. I had a dull headache that would not subside. It was maddening.

"What would cause this, doc?" I asked.

"We don't know exactly. Have you ever had weakness in your limbs or drop foot?" he asked.

"No, never—why?" I asked.

"Optic neuritits is often a precursor to multiple sclerosis," he said bluntly. I stared blankly at him, and he could see I did not know what he was referring to. "Here is some information that can better explain," he said, handing me some pamphlets. "I want to see you in a week. If anything gets worse, call the office immediately. For the next four days, I want you on 800 mg of ibuprofen."

I thanked him, made my follow-up appointment, and returned to my car.

Once in the car I started to read what he gave me. *This is not for real*, I thought. My mind raced as I read about multiple sclerosis. Confused and worried, I called my mom at work. She could tell I was upset, which made her upset.

"Let's go over everything tonight. There's probably nothing to worry about," she said, trying to reassure me.

On the drive home I couldn't help but think about my future. I was graduating from law school soon and ready to take on my next adventure.

Once home, I put the information away and went for a walk. I always felt better after I moved my body.

My mom came home a bit later. After giving me a big hug, she recommended that we leave a message for my eye doctor to talk with us tomorrow. I just wanted my headache to go away. I took my first dose of ibuprofen, and within thirty minutes my headache subsided. It was difficult, however, to read or watch television due to the issue with my vision.

I spent the next few days talking to doctors and doing as much research as my eye and head would allow. By the time a week went by, the ibuprofen had done its job. It reduced the inflammation in my optic nerve, restoring my sight and getting rid of the headache for good.

After walking out of the doctor's office, I never looked back. I tossed the information he handed me and went on with life. I did not think I would ever need it again.

THE SILENT FALL

When it happened again in 2002, at first I tried to ignore the pain and vision loss. I splashed water on my face, rubbed my eyes, and went for a run. But this time physical exertion seemed to make things worse. I immediately reached for the ibuprofen, and then told Steve what was going on. We were in the doctor's office the next afternoon. I underwent the same tests as in 1999, and I received the same results. With only three years between episodes, the doctor recommended I take the next step and seek out a doctor who treated patients with multiple sclerosis.

I kept telling myself that this was not happening. I was the owner of a new business, and I intended to see it through. I was determined to not let anything interfere with the life I was attempting to create. After MRIs, office visits to multiple doctors, and a spinal tap, the doctors all agreed that I should immediately go on medication. However, this was not your everyday medication. Beta interferons had to be injected intramuscularly, and it was guaranteed that if I did not take a pain reliever of some sort, I would feel like I had the flu. The doctors said I should prepare to alter my work week and my schedule.

I was angry; I just wanted the symptoms to disappear. *Nothing a few bottles of wine won't fix,* I thought. For the next several days I plowed through work like nothing was wrong. The ibuprofen helped to control the inflammation in my eye. I was bound and determined to get through this latest "thing," whatever this "thing" was. I worked hard during the day and drank my way through each evening.

Steve and I had a big learning curve to figure out. What exactly was multiple sclerosis? We scoured the Internet and attended support groups. I was not happy with any of the prognoses. I had been an athlete my entire life. I functioned at a level few people choose to or could as an agent, and I was not going to let this beat me.

After I iced my upper arm for ten minutes until it was numb and took 600 mg of ibuprofen, Steve administered the first injection. I could feel it in my muscle, and I asked Steve to push the plunger slowly. Then it was time to get comfortable and go to sleep.

The next morning I woke up and felt like a truck had run me over. My arm hurt, and my body was sluggish. I thought that drinking more coffee would do the trick, but no luck.

How in the world am I going to function at work like this? I thought. I took 800 mg of ibuprofen, dragged myself into the shower, then into the car, and finally into the sports performance center. I said a quick hello to my staff and then went into my office and closed the door. A few hours later I felt better. But half the day had gone by with not much accomplished.

I functioned this way for almost a year. Repeated MRIs showed no progression of the disease, which was great. But I was continuously irritated by the fact that I was losing a day's worth of productivity each week. As a result, my business began to suffer. My staff knew I had a health challenge, but I never informed them of the specifics. My head sports performance coach did his best to fill in the gaps in my absence, but without my ability to be fully engaged, we had a hard time making our numbers each month.

Steve and I had put all our savings into the business, and we were determined to see it through. But everything we tried seemed to fall short. One day we were faced with declaring bankruptcy or closing the facility and cutting our losses. After consulting with attorneys and family, we decided bankruptcy was not an option. We had lost more than $750,000 in the venture, and Steve was pouring every dime he made in his practice into the center. The corporate office offered no solutions, leaving us with major bills to pay as well as a severance package to our head performance coach.

One morning we called all of our staff into the conference room and broke the news. They were surprised but not shocked that we were closing our doors. What shocked them was my health status. For the first time I explained exactly what was going on, using the words *multiple sclerosis*. I wanted to crawl into a hole. I failed my mission.

For the next several months, Steve and I negotiated with the landlord. We paid off what we could and even sold some of the equipment to do so. I was angry at everything and everyone. I was tired of taking medication that made me sick, and I was tired of people telling me everything was going to be okay. I was desperate for solutions and continued to search for them.

One answer came in the form of a doctor who had an unconventional practice. After another round of clear MRIs, this doctor decided I should stop taking the beta interferons, against the recommendation of the other doctor who had prescribed them. It was one of the best decisions I could make. I began to feel better, and I was able to return to exercise.

But each morning when I woke up, I would ask myself, "Now what?" I had never failed at anything, and losing my business weighed heavily on me. It took me a long time to realize that losing my business was not a failure, but one of the greatest learning experiences of my life. I learned to evaluate my opportunities more strategically, and I learned to ask more quality questions of people and situations. I learned how to negotiate better, I learned to be more patient with myself and others, and most of all I learned to stop trying to hide all of the bad stuff from people and instead be vulnerable and committed to finding solutions. I also quit the "blame game." While I felt unsupported by our corporate offices, it was my fault that my business failed.

Eventually the legal matters were handled, and I moved on to my next adventure. The best part? After five years of clear MRI reports, it was determined that I had been misdiagnosed—I did not have MS!

In 2005, with a newfound hope and life skills I could use and pass on to others, I started my law enforcement career again—this time with the Montgomery County Department of Police in Montgomery County, Maryland. They were looking for a protection specialist to help lead the Executive Protection Division. I was their ideal candidate and a perfect fit. One of my partners was a former United States Secret Service Lieutenant in the Uniformed Division. We had an instant connection. I felt as though I had an advocate—someone who knew what "protection" was and who would back me up as we built the division.

This was different than the Secret Service. I was not a mere employee, part of a twenty-person squad. Although I was hired because of my experience as an agent, the Executive Protection Division was comprised of myself and three others. The four of us would be responsible for putting this division on the map, making recommendations and presenting our ideas to some of the highest-ranking officials in local government. We succeeded and became one of the most respected divisions in the police department.

With my marriage and career thriving, life was full and worth living again. And then, in July 2007, I faced my biggest challenge yet. Soon Steve and I would welcome a new person into our life, and suddenly I was scared again. Not of a thunderstorm or a dumpster crashing, but of my ability to stay present without turning to alcohol, which had been my crutch to "take the edge off" during previous times of stress.

This skinny little six-pound bundle of joy turned our well-ordered life upside down. On July 18, 2007, Steve and I became adoptive parents. When Steve and I married, we talked about having children. My sister and I were adopted. We are part of an extended family of adopted kids, and I shared with Steve that I would like to adopt.

Selfishly, I did not want to be confined to a desk for nine months. Truthfully, I was scared—I was a big chicken. I watched my sister's pregnancy and birth of my oldest nephew. It was an experience that, let's just say, confirmed that I had no interest in pushing a watermelon through my nostril. I knew that Steve and I could provide a loving home. After talking it over with Steve for more than a year, he became comfortable with the idea.

Our adoption process was not the typical one. We were referred to an adoption facilitator, and within a few weeks she put us in touch with a young mom who was trying to find a family for the baby boy she was carrying. On Father's Day 2007 she chose us to become her baby's parents. A short time later, we boarded a plane to San Diego, California. After a three-hour drive east to El Centro, we met our baby boy. We named him Hayden.

I was given three months off and quickly learned what caring for an infant demanded. With bottles every three hours, I thanked my lucky stars for the career I had chosen because I already knew how to quickly adjust to strategic napping.

My maternity leave went by quickly, and it was time to seek out childcare. My mom and sister stepped up until we could find a nanny. There were days when Hayden was asleep when I left for work and asleep when I returned home. I missed being with my son—those special times together in the rocking chair, watching him roll around on the floor, and even the way he smiled before spitting up after he finished a bottle.

Each evening I was on duty brought loneliness. Steve was at home with Hayden while I was at work. *Something is very wrong with this picture,* I thought. At times I found myself drifting back into my old ways. I would isolate myself and begin drinking again. I would catch myself starting to slip. When the alcohol ran out, I would promise myself I would stop, a promise I would break.

May 11, 2011, delivered news I had been waiting ten years to receive. I cried tears of joy and triumph along with so many others:

11:35 p.m. EDT
THE PRESIDENT: Good evening. Tonight, I can report to the American people and to the world that the United States has conducted an operation that killed Osama bin Laden,

the leader of al Qaeda, and a terrorist who was responsible for the murder of thousands of innocent men, women, and children.

It was nearly ten years ago that a bright September day was darkened by the worst attack on the American people in our history. The images of 9/11 are seared into our national memory—hijacked planes cutting through a cloudless September sky; the Twin Towers collapsing to the ground; black smoke billowing up from the Pentagon; the wreckage of Flight 93 in Shanksville, Pennsylvania, where the actions of heroic citizens saved even more heartbreak and destruction.

And yet we know that the worst images are those that were unseen to the world. The empty seat at the dinner table. Children who were forced to grow up without their mother or their father. Parents who would never know the feeling of their child's embrace. Nearly three thousand citizens taken from us, leaving a gaping hole in our hearts.

On September 11, 2001, in our time of grief, the American people came together. We offered our neighbors a hand, and we offered the wounded our blood. We reaffirmed our ties to each other, and our love of community and country. On that day, no matter where we came from, what God we prayed to, or what race or ethnicity we were, we were united as one American family.

We were also united in our resolve to protect our nation and to bring those who committed this vicious attack to justice. We quickly learned that the 9/11 attacks were carried out by al Qaeda—an organization headed by Osama bin Laden, which had openly declared war on the United States and was committed to killing innocents in our country and around the globe. And so we went to war against al Qaeda to protect our citizens, our friends, and our allies.

Over the last ten years, thanks to the tireless and heroic work of our military and our counterterrorism professionals, we've made great strides in that effort. We've disrupted terrorist attacks and strengthened our homeland defense . . .

Tonight, we give thanks to the countless intelligence and counterterrorism professionals who've worked tirelessly to achieve this outcome. The American people do not see their work, nor know their names. But tonight, they feel the satisfaction of their work and the result of their pursuit of justice.

We give thanks for the men who carried out this operation, for they exemplify the professionalism, patriotism, and unparalleled courage of those who serve our country. And they are part of a generation that has borne the heaviest share of the burden since that September day.

Finally, let me say to the families who lost loved ones on 9/11 that we have never forgotten your loss, nor wavered in our commitment to see that we do whatever it takes to prevent another attack on our shores.

And tonight, let us think back to the sense of unity that prevailed on 9/11. I know that it has, at times, frayed. Yet today's achievement is a testament to the greatness of our country and the determination of the American people.

The cause of securing our country is not complete. But tonight, we are once again reminded that America can do whatever we set our mind to. That is the story of our history,

> *whether it's the pursuit of prosperity for our people, or the struggle for equality for all our citizens; our commitment to stand up for our values abroad, and our sacrifices to make the world a safer place.*
>
> *Let us remember that we can do these things not just because of wealth or power, but because of who we are: one nation, under God, indivisible, with liberty and justice for all.*
>
> *Thank you. May God bless you. And may God bless the United States of America."*

These words ring the loudest in my head:

> *But tonight, we are once again reminded that America can do whatever we set our mind to. That is the story of our history, whether it's the pursuit of prosperity for our people, or the struggle for equality for all our citizens; our commitment to stand up for our values abroad, and our sacrifices to make the world a safer place.*

I began to ask myself: Was it time to forgive? Was it time for me to set my mind on something to help me grow as a person? Was it time to let go of being a victim who suffered because of the actions of a few evil men? Was it time to let go of being suspicious and cynical and trust again? Was it time to move on to the next challenge?

We had gone through several personnel changes within the

NEW BEGINNINGS

division, including a change of leadership at the top of the county. The new county executive we protected had a schedule that just would not quit and, to make matters worse, we found ourselves down a man in the division. This meant there were just three of us rotating days, nights, and weekends.

At times Steve and I were like two ships passing in the night. After working the night shift, Hayden and Steve would be already asleep when I got home. When I woke up the next morning, Steve would have already left for work, and our nanny would be with Hayden.

On the flip side, the day shift often had me up and out the door before Steve and Hayden woke up. By the time I returned home, I was stressed out and tired—and before I knew it, I was drinking before, during, and after dinner. One day I opened up the refrigerator to find the entire bottom shelf filled with beer. All I could do was sigh and hope that things would change. What I failed to realize was that the change I was looking for started with me.

One day I called a friend who I had not spoken to in a while. She was a very intuitive friend—you know, one of those friends that somehow senses exactly what is going on even without you saying much.

"When are you going to your first meeting, Sam?" she asked.

"What meeting? What are you talking about?" I replied.

"Your first AA meeting, Sam. I want you to call me after you go."

"I don't need—"

She cut me off mid-sentence. "Sam, stop trying to fool yourself. Find a meeting right now and then call me back," she ordered.

If there was one thing I knew how to do, it was to take orders—even from friends who I knew had my best interests in mind.

"Okay," I said; it was the only response I could muster.

My first AA meeting was uneventful. As I listened to people tell their stories, I felt like I did not belong. Being a law enforcement officer, I certainly did not know what being arrested for a DUI was like, nor did I relate to years spent in prison and living in halfway houses. So for the next few weeks, I sat in that meeting and hid everything about myself. If it came out that I was in law enforcement, I thought there would be a riot for sure.

Eventually I found a different AA group where I felt more comfortable. But I approached the twelve steps in a half-assed, halfhearted way. As a result I white-knuckled my way through a year and a half of sobriety. I was changing, though, and in turn things got better at work. A permanent nine-to-five position opened up, and I jumped at the opportunity.

In my new position I managed the Security Services Division of the police department and reported to the director. *Finally!* I thought. I got to see Steve and Hayden every morning and evening. I was now able to drop Hayden off at nursery school and go grocery shopping. Things were looking up.

My plan was to continue my career in this position until I retired. It's funny how things work out, however. Two months into my new assignment, the powers that be determined that I was too valuable an asset to remain in the Security Services Division; I was asked to return to the Executive Protection Division.

"So are you saying I was too good at my job protecting the county executive?" I asked the director and assistant chief.

NEW BEGINNINGS

"Yes, that's what we're saying, Sam. The division needs you back so things can run smoothly again," the assistant chief said.

I took a deep breath and shook my head. I looked at my director. "Are you serious about this? You know how long I waited for this assignment."

"I know, Sam. I'm sorry, but this is the way it has to be," he said.

My heart was breaking. All I could think about was how happy I was. How I finally felt like I could be there for Hayden and Steve. I was sad and angry all at once.

"I'll have to let you know my decision," I said to my director.

"No, Sam. You don't understand. This is going to happen. We don't need you to make a decision," was his response.

I left the office feeling as though this was all a dream. *How am I going to tell Steve?* I thought. I got into my car, and suddenly all kinds of questions flooded my brain.

How could they do this? Is there anything I can do to stop it? Why is this happening? How am I ever going to be a mom? What else am I going to have to give up? Is it time to move on?

When I got home that evening, I told Steve what had happened. I'm sure the neighbors down the street heard his response. He asked me what I wanted to do. I thought about Steve and how hard he worked. I thought about our plans for our family now that I was in a nine-to-five position. I thought about Hayden and the milestones I had missed. I also thought about myself. Not in a selfish way, but I thought about how I never included *me* in any decision making. I always sacrificed, no matter what the cost. And that cost was usually my well-being.

For a year Steve and I had been building a business on the side in the health and wellness field, and it was now bringing in some decent money. The compensation was almost enough to cover what I brought home each month minus the benefits. I thought about our long-term goals for this business and the positive difference it had already made in our lives.

A few days later I sat down at my computer and drafted my resignation letter. I had wasted enough time letting others dictate my worth in this world. It was time for Sam, Steve, and Hayden to spread our wings together and reach for our dreams.

Over the seven years I spent with the police department, I had helped several officers by sharing my story with them—my experiences during 9/11, my PTSD, and how I learned to use the tools I had been given. They saw me not as an unapproachable supervisor, but as a person who genuinely cared. I will always remember an experience with one officer in particular.

Several officers in my division had been in Iraq post 9/11. On one occasion I received a call at home one evening asking me to come in—one of the officers was having difficulty reporting to his assignment. Upon my arrival I immediately recognized the signs. He was pale and sweating, and his hands were trembling.

"Tell me what's going on, Kyle," I said, motioning for him to sit down next to me.

"It's all coming back, Lieu. I don't know why. I'm having nightmares, I can't sleep or eat, and I'm getting headaches."

I leaned forward and looked at him in the eyes. "Kyle, I know what you're going through. I've been there. I promise you, you are safe. No one can hurt you here. You are in charge at all times. You have to breathe."

Kyle took a deep breath. I handed him some water. He stared vacantly at the blank computer screen. A tear rolled down his cheek.

I put my hand on his arm. "Kyle, stay with me, bud." My touch brought him back to the present.

"I'm sorry, Lieutenant," he said, looking down at the floor.

"You don't have to apologize," I replied. I noticed color starting to return to his cheeks. "Take the rest of the shift off. Go home and text me when you get there."

"But I don't want to let you down or have the other guys talk about me," he said.

"You are not letting me down. As for the other guys . . ." I leaned in close so I could whisper, making sure no one else heard me. "Some of them are going through the same thing you are. They don't want anyone to know either."

I leaned back in my chair and looked at Kyle. His entire expression had changed to one of relief.

"Really, Lieu?"

"Really, Kyle. Go on home and call me when you get there. I'll see you tomorrow."

Okay, Lieutenant. Thank you."

"You're welcome, Kyle. You can call me anytime."

Being able to encourage and support these valiant men was some of my best work; it was what I valued most, and it was what I would miss the most. I had given everything I had to my law enforcement career. It was a career that brought chaos, fulfillment, devotion, and change—all for the betterment of those who I served.

TEN

THE ANSWER

SO THERE I was: no longer connected to any law enforcement agency, free to assume the responsibilities of building our health and wellness business, and serving my family as a full-time wife and mom. Every day brought a new adventure with Hayden. I was finally home.

I learned a lot throughout my law enforcement career. From agent to supervisor, I learned the skills it took to be successful at my job, but more importantly I learned about people. I learned to never quit and never stop growing. There is an air of invincibility when you go out into the world each day with a gun and a badge strapped to you. That invincibility was tested on 9/11 and almost toppled during my struggle with PTSD.

If I had quit the struggle, I would not be here. Hayden would have grown up without a mom, Steve without a wife, my mom without a daughter—you get the picture. I also would have given up on a learning process that healed me, strengthened my resolve, and exposed me to new and meaningful things. I would not trade my experience with PTSD for anything. It happened so that I could ultimately assist others.

When Steve and I started our health and wellness business in 2011, we met some interesting people. They were all entrepreneurs with a vision to change the future. The thing that stood out most to me was that the top leaders had all been through hell and back. Whether they had conquered illness, financial disasters, or debilitating accidents, or had been innocent victims of horrific childhood crimes perpetrated against them, these leaders all had made the decision to stop being victims of their own stories. They took a stand and faced their fears head on.

In their presence, I felt as though I was home; I had the sense that I had finally met people who understood me at my core. I wanted to know how they overcame their challenges. I wanted to know what books they read, what they studied, who they learned from, and how they became successful. I started to train with them as I began to create an income alongside my law enforcement career.

Over time these partners became my friends, and we traveled together. I immersed myself in the learning process. It wasn't so much learning how to do the business—it was learning about myself. For instance, ever since 9/11 I would let things go when they got too hard. I would let myself off the hook by saying, "I guess it wasn't meant to be." The Sam that used to dive into a learning challenge was now learning challenged. I did not understand it, nor did I like it.

I read everything my new friends recommended. I immersed myself in the writings of Tony Robbins, Darren Hardy, Dale Carnegie, Og Mandino, Dr. Henry Cloud, Robert Kiyosaki, and others. With each new book, I was reading *my story*. No, these self-empowerment giants hadn't been stricken with PTSD, but

THE ANSWER

they suffered and struggled in other ways—and they survived to tell their stories and impact the lives of others.

Through reading countless books and attending seminars, events, and webinars, the drive to learn, grow, and ultimately teach returned. With it came the ability to ask myself more quality questions. I used to wonder why I was different than everyone else. Why I could not just "half-ass" my way through life. Why I was given so much pain and suffering to endure. The answer did not come until November 1, 2015—until I had moved more than 1,300 miles from where I used to call home.

❦

After leaving law enforcement, I had more time to pursue our health and wellness business. Steve, on the other hand, was coming home from work more and more frustrated. While the additional income we were bringing in helped us do special things together, the joy was short-lived due to the stresses and demands his office placed on him. Whether it was the landlord, electronic billing, processing insurance claims, or the ever-revolving door of training front desk staff, the chiropractic career he once loved was becoming a burden, and he began talking about finding another way to make a living.

We also were both growing tired of the winter season in Maryland, which seemed to be growing longer with each passing year. I happened to travel to Dallas for some of my training, an area that held fond memories for me. It was at the Dallas Field Office of the United States Secret Service that I received my most amusing briefing as I headed out to then-President Bush's ranch in Crawford, Texas. I'll never forget the senior agent telling us, "Watch out for the tarantulas!" The people, the climate, the vast wide-open spaces, and the slower pace of life stuck with me every time I returned to the hustle and bustle of busy New York City.

One day Steve came home and said, "I'm ready." At first I thought he was talking about being ready for dinner since he caught me off-guard working at my desk. But seeing the look on his face, I asked, "Ready for what?"

"Let's do it. Let's get out of here. I'm ready to sell my practice," he said.

"Are you serious?" I responded. He had mentioned the possibility before, but I could sense that this time he had really hit the wall. In fact, he had already reached out to a lawyer to discuss the process of selling his practice. It was a relatively simple process if he had a buyer.

"Let's move somewhere south, somewhere much warmer," he said.

Over the next few months, as Steve worked on putting his practice up for sale, I explored some possibilities. We looked at Virginia, Georgia, and Florida. We both knew we wanted a house on the water.

A few weeks later I happened to be once again in Dallas for some special business training. There was a realtor in our group, and I asked him to show me some properties located on two large man-made lakes. As we drove from property to property, I was astounded by the low cost of real estate. The homes were two to three times the size of our townhome for a fraction of the price.

When I returned home, I asked Steve what he thought about putting Texas on the list—specifically Dallas.

"Dallas? I want trees and water!" he exclaimed.

After I stopped laughing, I showed him the real estate listings with pictures of the properties I had visited.

"These can't be the prices, Sam. There's no way," he said.

"Yes, those are the prices for waterfront property, Steve. These are all current listings. Howard took me to see them," I responded.

Steve was speechless. He immediately went to the computer and double- and triple-checked the prices.

"Holy cow, Sam. I can't believe it! When can we go back so I can see them?"

We planned a family trip to Dallas in December 2012. Hayden was on Christmas break from school, and we stayed with some friends. We visited each property, along with some others that had just come on the market. The day before we were to return home, we visited a property on Lake Ray Hubbard in Rockwall. The house had been recently renovated. There was a pool and a huge backyard with a paved path leading to a boat dock, complete with jet-ski lifts.

"This is going to be my room, Mommy and Daddy," Hayden announced. It was the only house we'd seen that he reacted to. He also could not wait to swim in the pool. Neither Steve nor I had ever owned property like this. We fell in love with it, just like Hayden.

The following February, on Valentine's Day, we signed the papers and closed on our new home. It is our own slice of heaven, and I wake up each day grateful for what we have.

Soon enough, however, the new stresses of home ownership and trying to build a business in a new zip code reactivated that familiar feeling of needing to "take the edge off." Whether it was the pool requiring service, Hayden needing help at school, the phone ringing incessantly, or replacing appliances, taking the edge off was the proverbial "monkey on my back," and it followed me to my new home. I started drinking, stopped, and started again several times. The experts call this "playing with fire."

By September 2014 I had dug myself a hole so deep that once again I was morally and spiritually bankrupt. I was risking everything I had—my family, my friendships, my business, my very life. The lessons I had thought I'd learned back in 2011 were now so deeply buried that I could no longer see the greatness inside of me.

One day I went on a bender, and in the middle of it, I knew I was ready to give up. I called a friend, who somehow convinced me to get in a cab and come to her house. When I arrived she pulled me inside and shut the door. I sat on the floor of her office and then passed out. Later she helped me up off the floor, and we ended up in her backyard.

I wanted to crawl into a hole, but she would not let me. She grabbed the sunglasses I was wearing and got right in my face. She literally forced me to face my fears, and it rocked me sober. Every time I tried to look away out of shame, she would grab my face and force me to look at her.

She called Steve, and he joined us. I couldn't bear to look at Steve. I had let him down again. I knew this was my very last chance. I needed help—and fast.

The next day I drove three hours south to Austin to stay with a friend who was a trauma specialist and familiar with EMDR. She also had been sober for twenty-plus years. A week away from home and the intensive treatment helped me identify triggers I had held onto ever since 9/11. It was hard for me to believe that something that happened thirteen years ago could still affect me so strongly.

I learned that cortisol, the stress hormone, carried markers through my body. As it continued its flow, a thought, a feeling, a smell—anything at all—could trigger a stress response in me. So although I had not experienced any nightmares, flashbacks, or anything else that caused me to return to "that day," the cortisol release in my body was enough to cause me to reach for a drink, or two, or ten.

It came down to a choice. Did I want to learn how to handle the stress, or did I want to "check out"? If I chose the latter, I knew I would be divorced, and I would never see my friends again.

Now, you might be thinking, *She's not dealing with anything anyone else does not deal with on any given day,* and you would be absolutely correct. The difference is that on 9/11, my body's chemistry changed, and "normal," everyday stressors caused a flight-or-fight response in me, something most people don't experience.

I returned home with new tools in my toolbox and a renewed vision of what my future could be when I used, trusted, and believed in those tools. During the remainder of 2014, I made it a point to reread the motivational books that had expanded my mind and given me a vision for how I wanted to live and what kind of contribution I wanted to make. I found a local AA group and started working the twelve steps, this time wholeheartedly. With Steve focused on the business, which was providing a steady income for us, I could focus on getting well.

We rang in 2015 together with friends. I felt as though I

had a new beginning, a clean slate to work from and build on. Before I knew it, I had completed the twelve steps. Reenergized and refocused, I joined Steve in growing our business, and I made a conscious intention to attend every single school event with Hayden. I learned that living life with intention provided a much richer experience than approaching it aimlessly. It's the difference between having a simple cup of coffee from a diner and taking the time to grind the beans, boil the water, and allow it to steep in a French press before enjoying a thick, rich decadent cup. Who would not want to enjoy the French press-brewed coffee every day?

Part of living intentionally meant creating goals. A big goal for me was to take the summer and go on a travel adventure. After all, Texas is a lot bigger than Maryland, and I wanted to see our new home state. We rented a cabin in Terlingua and hiked for miles in the Big Bend National Park. It was incredible—nature's majesty at its best. The glorious sunrises were rivaled only by the magnificent sunsets. Connecting to nature this way strengthened our relationship.

As summer turned to fall, I carried that trip with me and made it a point to bond with nature every day. I moved my newfound meditation time outdoors under our covered patio. Rain or shine, from six to seven every morning, that's where you'll find me. Being aware of and connected to that which is greater than myself allowed me to create a space for gratitude, and I experienced a comfort level I had not felt in a long time. I would rely on that sense of well-being heavily with September 11, 2015, right around the corner.

THE ANSWER

September 11, 2015, was a Friday, which meant memorial and remembrance services would be held throughout the weekend. I has planned to do what I had done each year after 9/11: enjoy a quiet day at home reflecting on the blessings I was fortunate to have been granted.

My cell phone rang. It was one of the Texas state representative's staff members. She contacted me after reading an article about me in the local paper to request that I participate in a special remembrance service nearby.

At first I was surprised. *This must be a very connected state representative,* I thought. Being around the political scene for so many years, I was used to politicians showing up at different events for no other reason than to make sure people noticed they were there so as to secure votes in the next election. This request was different.

The staff member explained that the representative was a huge supporter of law enforcement, and he wanted to make sure people did not forget the sacrifices of the first responders on 9/11. He was not sure how to do that until he read my story. I agreed to participate and reached out to the main contact for the event.

"You are a gift from God!" said the voice on the other end of the phone. I did not know how to respond.

"I . . . um . . . wow . . . thank you," was all that came out of my mouth.

"I prayed last night that a survivor of 9/11 would be revealed and participate in our service," he said.

"I would be honored," I responded. He went on to explain what the event was about, and at the end of our conversation, he asked if I would speak to all the volunteers who were making the service possible. I agreed.

After we hung up, my heart begin to race. *I'm really doing this,* I thought. It had been fourteen years since I had told my story, with the exception of a few friends, a small local Rotary group, and the local newspaper. I certainly had never shared it in front of a large group of people. I told Steve the news, and he was excited and happy for me.

As I continued with my quiet day, flipping through the channels on the TV, I stopped on the History Channel, which was broadcasting the events of 9/11. I took a deep breath and decided to watch.

"Oh my God," I said out loud. I had just heard the answer to a question I held onto for fourteen years: What was the sound I heard in the elevator? An engineer explained that when American Airlines Flight 11 crashed into the north tower, it was full of jet fuel. When it exploded, the jet fuel poured out of the plane and down the elevator shafts; it was the roar of the fire I heard barreling toward us—like a freight train. "Everything in the shaft would have been on fire," he said.

"Everything in the shaft would have been on fire." The words roared through my head over and over. I felt as though I might be having a heart attack. I had not been on fire. The elevator car had not caught fire. *How?* I thought. *How is this possible? I am here, and I was not on fire.*

I walked outside, fell to my knees, and looked up to the sky. "Thank you. Thank you," I said as the tears started to flow. I walked back into the house, where Steve was in his office. He looked up from the computer. "Are you okay?" he asked. I told him what

I had just heard. I held onto him tightly and cried. None of the evidence presented could explain why I had not been consumed by a giant fireball that day.

I closed my eyes. At that moment I felt as though everything in the universe had shifted. The newspaper article, the phone call, watching this particular television channel.

What is the message here, God? I prayed.

On Sunday, September 13, 2015, I addressed fifty volunteers and their family members. There were law enforcement officers, firefighters, military personnel, and state and county officials, as well as those who traveled from Oklahoma. I thanked them for their service, their hard work, and for not forgetting the victims—those that died and those who were still here to bear witness. I shared a quote from John Updike:

Suddenly summoned to witness something great and horrendous, we keep fighting not to reduce it to our own smallness.

When the service concluded, I knew no one here would ever stop fighting. They would never reduce 9/11 to just another day. I was proud to call these people my brothers and sisters. I had just met them, but they understood. They understood the pain, the grief, the sacrifice. And they understood what it meant to remember.

The remainder of the day was filled with hugs and thank yous. The state representative was humble, gracious, and direct in his commentary.

I so love Texas, I thought. I spent the evening quietly thinking about the day's events and the new friends I had made. I could not help but think of the words *bear witness*. They swirled in my head until I calmly fell asleep.

The next morning, I woke up unusually early. I made a hot cup of coffee and went outside, where I sat in silence. It was just me, the moon, and the stars. I closed my eyes and asked, "What is it you want me to do?"

I went to our guest room closet, where I dug out some old Secret Service memories from a box I had stored there. I came across the *People* magazine from 9/11, as well as the special 9/11 edition of *The Secret Service Star,* an internal publication. As I flipped through the pages and looked at the pictures, I reflected again on the remembrance service and the words *bear witness*.

"What am I supposed to do?" I asked myself. I had been journaling for a while and began rereading some of the entries. The majority of the entries had the word *serve* or *service* in them. *Hmm,* I thought.

Finishing my coffee, I went back inside; it was time to get our son ready for school. As the next few days went by, I found myself asking the same question repeatedly, "What do you want me to do?" That same word, *serve*, kept coming to me. How would I serve? More importantly, who would I serve?

What I stumbled into was completely unexpected. I began reading survival stories from current and former military members, police officers, firefighters, and other first responders. Their stories were compelling and heart-wrenching. Every one of them mentioned PTSD. They were telling their stories so others would not forget.

I felt as though some invisible force was moving inside me.

THE ANSWER

I sat down at my computer, opened a blank Word document, and started typing everything I could remember. It was a jumbled mess, but I didn't let that stop me. The result was the humble beginning of this book, and it led me to find deeper answers the questions about how and whom I would serve.

◆

I continued my new ritual of starting each day outside in the quiet hours of the morning, Undisturbed, I could "hear" what was being spoken to me. I kept journaling. "Why me?" was still the biggest question I had. All those years of torment and torture—there had to be a reason. I knew I was put on this planet to serve, but why? And where?

On November 1, 2015, I was invited to a special church service to hear a Vietnam veteran tell his story of survival. A phosphorous grenade had exploded in his hand, burning over 90 percent of his body. He was not expected to survive, but he did. "My biggest question was why? Why me, God?" he said.

I snapped to attention in my seat. My heart began to pound, and I began to sweat.

"Because God could trust me with the scars."

Tears welled up in my eyes; I squeezed Steve's hand tightly. *Because God could trust me with the scars.* "Thank you, God," I said silently. At that moment I felt as though a five-hundred-pound weight was lifted from my shoulders. I had my answer.

A few days later I came across a picture of a piece of art that moved me. Human hands formed the shape of a heart, and the hands were painted to look like the American flag. Words like *heart, patriot,* and *healing* came to mind. The idea for Heroes 4 Healing, an outreach group that would serve first responders, police, fire, and military personnel, was born.

As with any new idea, I had doubts. But stronger than those doubts, I had belief—and I embraced it. I began meeting people who were eager to help and had stories to share—individuals who had suffered with PTSD or were in the thick of it and looking for help. None of this was accidental.

Heroes 4 Healing launched on January 19, 2016—a very special day: my fourteenth wedding anniversary. With everything I learned from my experience with PTSD, I wanted to provide a safe place where people could come and listen to stories of how others recovered from whatever trauma had thrust them into the darkness.

I wanted to make the biggest impact with as little documentation or red tape as possible. I had heard too many stories of people seeking help from professionals they thought they could trust, and in the process labels of PTSD or "unfit to return to duty" became part of their official file. This created was a significant level of anger, resentment, and distrust in the system that was supposed to be helping them. They were left to suffer in silence again.

I heard a story of a young soldier who spent ten years devoted to serving his country. He loved what he did. After returning from the second tour in Afghanistan, he became withdrawn and angry. One of his friends recommended that he get some help. He valued his friend's opinion and saw someone he thought he could trust. When he put in for his third tour with his unit, his request was denied. The person from whom he sought help had put PTSD in his file, which prevented him from returning to duty. Rather than helping him get well, they told him he could either change units—which meant leaving the friends he had done battle with, bled with, and cried with—or he could be medically discharged. "What a shitty decision," was the way he described it.

I wanted Heroes 4 Healing to avoid this type of situation, so it could truly be a trusted place for those who came to us. Heroes 4 Healing offers peer-to-peer support in a confidential setting for current and former members of the U.S. Military, law enforcement, firefighters, and first responders without any paper trail. This means people can come and openly share what they are struggling with without judgment or having to worry about being labeled. So far we have worked with Vietnam veterans, EMS workers, former police officers, federal agents, and members of the military. The common thread we all share is that PTSD does not discriminate, and the road to getting well starts with sharing our voices so we can all heal as a community.

ELEVEN

LESSONS FOR LIFE

I LEARNED MANY lessons on my way to getting well and being back in the proverbial saddle. It was a journey that allowed me to return to myself. If you are dealing with something in your life that has derailed you and taken you away from the magnificent person you are, I hope the following six lessons will assist you to gain a new perspective.

1) Exercise your soul and body.

> *All I have seen teaches me to trust*
> *the Creator for all I have not seen.*
> —Ralph Waldo Emerson

Whatever your belief system might be, having faith in something bigger than us and trusting that it is guiding us to be bigger than our circumstances is key.

I will never forget the day I lost my faith. I consciously chose to give it up because I mistakenly believed that our Supreme Being allowed 9/11 to happen, that He purposely put me where He did to hurt me, that He allowed my grandfather to die at a time when I still needed him in my life. I was naïve, and instead of asking key questions of my spiritual leaders, I turned my back on everything good, on what could have kept me "present." I closed myself off until that fateful night when I tried to "check out." That night, when I could not pull the trigger, His voice spoke to me, and I realized I was meant to live, that I was meant to do something more. Somehow I knew I was meant to rise above my circumstances and do something with the scars He trusted me with.

How does this happen? How does one choose to reconnect with his or her faith?

It is a conscious choice. We can choose to hold fast to the idea that there is something bigger out there that has created a journey unique to us—a journey that will help us grow and be better than we were yesterday. I have never met anyone who has not struggled to get where he or she is. The question of how is answered when we choose to do things that bring us closer to our higher power, whatever you choose to call it.

Here is a simple list of activities I do each day. I challenge you to try them if you are not doing them already. It will take you places you did not expect.

Each morning I read something positive for five to ten minutes. It may be a book of affirmations or positive messages, or something that I want to learn.

Next I go outside (or to a very quiet place if I am traveling) and sit quietly with my eyes closed for ten to twenty minutes. I thank God for granting me another day on this earth, and I think about what I am grateful for. I visualize myself achieving my goals, and I ask Him to bless my journey. I call this my meditation time. You may call it your quiet time or reflection time or whatever you like. The whole point is to ground yourself in a positive place so you can focus on the greater things in store for your life.

I then journal about everything I have been shown. It is extraordinary to look back through my journals and reflect on all the goals I have achieved—goals for myself individually and for my family, my health, my finances, and my spirituality.

Exercise is another key component. I make sure to move for at least thirty minutes a day. My workouts vary. In general I pick two days out of the week to do cardio, and I do high-intensity weight work on the other three days, with two days off for rest and recovery.

I highly recommend including a weight and strength component. First, it burns more calories and second, it is a challenge—and we grow by challenging ourselves. The options are endless. Kettlebells, sandbags, and free weights are all there for you to take advantage of.

The entire process should take you around ninety minutes. Now, I know what you are thinking. *I don't have that kind of time in the morning, Sam!* Granted, some people don't. I suggest that you do your reading, meditation/reflection time, and journaling in one chunk. If it's five minutes for each thing, then start with that. Try getting up a few minutes earlier—nothing extreme—and you will find it gets easier and easier. In fact, I predict that you will reach a point where you will never want to miss it!

Exercise can come later in the day if necessary. The goal is to be committed to yourself. We often put others before ourselves. Why? Because we were taught that doing for ourselves is selfish. I can promise you this: If you make the commitment to yourself and do the things I have outlined, by giving to yourself each morning, you will be able to give to so many others along your journey that it will astound you.

2) Choose belief.

> *Believing in yourself is not a luxury.*
> *It is where the wildness enters your genius;*
> *the deepest revolution possible.*
> *—Rachel Wolchin*

In my experience, it is easier to stay angry and grow cold, callous, and even suspicious after a trauma. Have you ever heard someone say, "It's easier to focus on the negative than the positive?" It's true. Keep track of how many times you complain as you go through your day. I bet you will find a lot more things in the negative column than the positive. The longer we stay in that negative place, though, the harder it is to regain our belief in the positive. Why? Because belief in yourself, in others, in a power that created everything for your benefit, cannot live in a negative state.

During my struggle with PTSD, it was so much easier to stay "checked out" at the bottom of a bottle than face the complexities of life. I hated what was happening to me, and I chose to believe that I was a victim. I lost my belief in anything good.

Have you ever heard the saying, "What you speak about, you bring about"? I spoke words of defeat, anger, and worthlessness to myself, and it took me to a place in my mind that I never want to visit again.

LESSONS FOR LIFE

Deep down inside we all sense that there is something greater than ourselves out there. Think of how you feel when you:

- watch a beautiful sunrise or sunset
- attend a sporting event where your team totally "crushes it"
- listen to your kids laugh with pure joy
- visit a beautiful place
- read something that moves you so much you can feel it in your heart

The more of these experiences we have, the more we bind the positive emotions they generate to our souls, empowering us to believe in what is good and right with the world. These strong feelings create our belief.

Perhaps, though, you grew up in a home where you were constantly criticized or told you would never amount to anything. Maybe those are the beliefs you have about yourself. You feel worthless, angry, defeated, as though nothing good ever happens to you.

I had some of those beliefs after 9/11. When I realized that I had made a decision to stay in the emotions of those negative beliefs, I finally realized I could also choose to focus on the belief that there were better days yet to come. After stringing together first two, then three, four, and five better days during which I focused on the special people and things I had in my life, things got better. I focused on my little boy, my husband, my dog, the way the cool autumn breeze felt, the simple joys that were mine—and the desire to believe in myself returned. Based on these things, I could distinguish what was good and bad, positive and negative, and I consciously chose to believe in the good.

3) Overcome fear.

> *Fear defeats more people than*
> *any other one thing in the world.*
> *—Ralph Waldo Emerson*

After the events of 9/11, I thought that if I was fearful of something, it meant I should not do it. My definition of *fear* was an acronym: "Forget Everything And Run." I was a master at this. I set up each day around this definition. I ran until I could not run anymore because I had imprisoned myself in my own house. I was completely defeated.

When I started EMDR therapy, I was introduced to another acronym: "Face Everything And Rise." I began to ask myself quality questions such as, "What kind of life could I have if I put my fears aside?" and "What could I accomplish if I wasn't scared anymore?"

I remembered what frightened me during my Secret Service training. Two memories in particular kept coming back. The first was jumping from a ten-meter platform into a pool. It was a mandatory part of our training, and we all had to do it. I had never gone near a high dive as a kid. I never jumped off the cliffs into the lake at summer camp. I guess I had heard of too many people getting hurt and decided I was never going to do something like that voluntarily. However, nothing at the Secret Service Training Center was voluntary.

My turn came; there was no turning back. I had to do it or I would fail, which would mean the premature end of my career. I remember walking to the edge with my heart pounding. I crossed my arms, closed my eyes, and . . . *splash!*

The second memory was the first building entry we had to perform as a team. We wore body armor and used simunition rounds (paint-filled bullets) in our duty weapons. The simunition rounds would exit our weapons with the same velocity as the regular .357 rounds we used. We were all scared and sweating so much we could barely grip our weapons.

"Police!" the front man yelled.

Bam! The halogen tool took out the front door.

"Police! Stop! Let me see your hands!" we yelled, seeing the instructor who was playing the part of the bad guy at the top of the stairs.

Pop! Pop! Pop! The bullets started flying. I took two to my body armor, one in my arm and one in my leg. The bruises lasted for weeks.

It was one of the craziest, scariest, and amazing training exercises we experienced. A little known fact about the Secret Service is that we served our own search warrants. The skills learned in the building entry training were critical. In New York we executed many building entries, and I am happy to report that no one was ever injured or shot. In almost all of the raids, we confiscated firearms and sometimes drugs.

During my EMDR therapy, as I remembered these experiences, I thought, *If I could do this, I could work through, face anything, and rise.* That is exactly what I chose to do. Week after week my EMDR therapy took me back to the scary places in my mind that paralyzed me with fear, and together my therapist and I worked through them. The therapy allowed me to put fear in its proper place and eventually restored my sense of accomplishment.

I learned how to deal with my fear—how to compartmentalize it and rise above it. A friend shared a verse from the Bible with me that says it best: "God did not give us a spirit of timidity and fear, but of power and of love and of a sound mind" (2 Timothy 1:7).

Choose to face the things that frighten you most, and move through them with determination. Find peace in knowing you are not the only one scared right now. Grab onto the people who believe in you, and you too will find the courage to face your fears and rise.

4) Be courageous.

You gain strength, courage, and confidence by every experience in which you really stop to look fear in the face.
You are able to say to yourself, "I lived through this horror.
I can take the next thing that comes along."
—Eleanor Roosevelt

I believe we are all born with courage. As newborns we know nothing of fear. Fear is learned from the negatives life throws at us. All the while our courage lurks in the background. It beckons us to act. It's the angst you feel when something happens that you know you have to face—that twinge in your gut that says, "You have to do this, no matter what." Having the courage to face what frightens you most will take you places you have only dreamed of. And it all starts with a choice.

There were many days I did not want to get out of bed, let alone go to my EMDR appointments. The therapy brought me back to the places I feared most, the places that caused me to cower, to shrink away from my former self. Sometimes after an appointment, I would rush home and seek solace in my darkened bedroom where I felt safe.

Would I ever have the courage to do the things I used to do? was a question that haunted me. Everything I had done up to this point, however, was exactly what I needed to focus on, because everything I accomplished had required action. Without deciding to take action to put my life back on track, I realized that I would remain fearful and full of doubt.

Finally I resigned myself to the pain and let my excuses go, just as I had experienced during training. I knew that continuing my therapy would leave me temporarily bruised. It was no different than the physical bruises I came home with after getting tossed around in the mat room or shot with simunitions. The bruises healed, and I became stronger and wiser with each bold new step I took into the unknown.

When my therapy was complete, I could see that life was going to take me in a very different direction. I was armed with the courage that no matter what, I was going to make it. I could never have imagined that the destination would have so many twists and turns. But the journey through the hard stuff is rarely a straight one, and it is in the valleys where we find the courage to grow and learn. We may cry or want to tear our hair out, but then we succeed.

5. Take action.

> *Knowing is not enough, we must apply.*
> *Willing is not enough, we must do.*
> —Bruce Lee

Simply knowing something without applying it can be compared to sitting still as the world passes by. I had to learn that my struggle was actually my greatest asset. I had played the victim so well for so many years. I had allowed my fears to keep me from learning and taking action. When I found my courage and came to a point where I decided to stop playing the victim, I took on new challenges at work and in my personal life. I had to learn new skills and then apply them.

In the police department I was asked to take on all of the administrative duties and contract oversight for our division. I had no idea what that meant—but it allowed me to be home each evening with my family, something I had not been able to do for years. It required me to meet new people and rely on my sergeants for guidance on a few projects. Can you imagine a lieutenant looking to her sergeants for answers? Isn't it supposed to be the other way around? I learned to determine the best course of action—whether at work or with a personal decision—by consulting with those who had been there before. After gaining the requisite knowledge, I could then act.

As I continue to embrace personal development, I am nuts about the action part of things. That's why I am very strategic about what I choose to learn. I always ask myself a single question before I begin: "Will this course, webinar, book, or conference bring me closer to my goals right now?" If the answer is yes, I run with it, focusing all my energies on it and taking all the necessary actions. By doing, I learn, and once I learn, I know. If the answer is no, I move on.

I want to stop here and emphasize an important point: Having a singular focus is key. Singularly focus on one course, one webinar, one success coach. Just as I did with my EMDR treatment, I focus on one thing until successful. I have learned that this is how the brain thrives best.

Thanks to book *The One Thing* by Gary Keller, I've learned that multitasking is a myth and something we should avoid. When you try to do too many things, nothing gets done. Whether you are new to personal development or not, I challenge you to take the next ninety days and focus on *one thing*—whether it's a book or online course—that will bring you closer to your goals.

6. Persevere no matter what.

> *Courage and perseverance have a magical talisman,*
> *before which difficulties disappear*
> *and obstacles vanish into air.*
> —*John Quincy Adams*

If you take nothing away from this chapter, I hope you hide John Quincy Adams' words in your heart. To persevere despite your current situation is what will get you through anything. Giving up is too easy. When I was at my lowest point, I was looking for the easy way because it seemed that everything else I was facing was just too hard. I was tired, and I had lost the sense of who I was. I was focusing on how bad I felt instead of on the amazing things I had accomplished in my life.

I will never forget the night my higher power spoke to me. I knew I was meant to persevere and look beyond my current situation. But how? As I took action to get well, the how came. I decided to turn every day into a blessing by saying two simple words: "Thank you." Yes, it was that easy. Even now, as I move into new ventures, I start my day with a simple "Thank you" as a reminder of what I have overcome.

Perseverance is a huge key to survival, period. That, and a belief that you are meant to live a full life, bravely and fearlessly, is a winning combination that can take you to new heights.

EPILOGUE

WE CANNOT BE a nation that forgets. Recently I have seen a return to divisiveness, our United States torn apart because of a lack of leadership. But we do not have to buy into the "game." I believe that forgiveness is the key. Forgiveness doesn't excuse a wrongdoer's behavior. Forgiveness prevents that behavior from destroying your own heart.

In 2015 I decided to forgive Mohammad Atta for what he did. I also decided that in order to do that I had to return to the scene of his trespasses against our nation, his trespasses against me. His face haunted me night after night. For so long I fooled myself into thinking I could drink him away. He remained the last thing I held onto. I knew that in order to be "free" I had to let go.

As the train pulled away from the Newark station, the new Manhattan skyline came into view. I fixed my attention on the Freedom Tower, now called 1 WTC. I could feel my heart starting to pound. I took a deep breath and fought back tears. I put on my sunglasses and hugged Steve's arm. It had been fourteen years, five months, and twenty-five days since 9/11.

The night before my return to Ground Zero was surprisingly peaceful. I slept relatively well and exited the subway, prepared to step onto the hallowed ground, now a beautiful memorial to

THE SILENT FALL

the victims and survivors and a museum. I walked to the first reflecting pool. It was built on the exact site of where 2 WTC used to be. The name of every person who was killed is engraved in the brass railings which surround the pool.

Just keep breathing, Sam, I repeated to myself over and over again. As I looked down into the reflecting pool, my son took my hand. "Mom, why are all these names here?" he asked.

As I started to answer, I choked up. I couldn't speak. I motioned to Steve for help. He acted swiftly, answering Hayden's question and putting his arm around me. We stood there quietly hugging each other. I was not prepared to go to the 1 WTC reflecting pool yet, so we entered the museum.

The museum iss filled with artifacts. I saw twisted steel columns from both towers and the actual staircase that took many survivors from the WTC Plaza to Vesey Street below. I used those stairs almost daily. There were burned-out fire trucks from Engine Companies 3 and 7 and an ambulance.

The museum has an enclosed exhibit that chronicles 9/11 with video and personal items from survivors and victims. At first I was hesitant to enter, but a museum volunteer encouraged me to go in. "With what you went through, you may find it difficult, but I think you'll appreciate what the museum has created," she said.

With that I entered, Steve and Hayden by my side. We heard a rush of sirens and banging and voices being played through speakers, effectively conveying the chaos of 9/11. I moved quickly, trying to find a quieter place. I had a responsibility to protect Hayden from the most graphic pictures. Steve took on the responsibility of protecting me from some of the more graphic video presentations. As we moved through the exhibit, no one spoke. Some people cried, others sat quietly on benches, trying to comprehend what they were seeing. In one section of the exhibit, I saw a picture of one of my fellow Secret Service agents. "Hayden, come here," I said, as I motioned for him to join me.

"Mommy used to work with this man. His name is Tommy."

"Wow. He is rescuing that lady, isn't he, Mom?" Hayden asked.

"Yes, he is, Hayden. Tommy is a hero," I said as I fought back tears. I felt a sense of pride that the museum had chosen to include a picture of one of my colleagues.

We continued to walk through the exhibit. At 12:37 p.m., I stood before a picture of Mohammad Atta's face. I stared into his black eyes—the eyes of evil that had haunted me for years. I was angry. "Steve, could you please take Hayden?" I asked.

Steve and Hayden disappeared around the next corner. I took a deep breath. "You fucking son of a bitch," I said under my breath, my heart racing. I closed my eyes and took another deep breath. As I stood there with my eyes closed, I remembered all the beautiful things that had come into my life since 9/11. I focused on my son's face and what God had put into my heart. I could feel HIS presence surrounding me. I felt safe. As my heart rate slowed, I opened my eyes and stared back into Mohammad Atta's eyes. "You will not have one more minute of my life. I forgive you," I whispered.

Immediately I felt as if a huge weight was lifted from my shoulders. "I forgive you," I repeated.

I was free.

I left the museum and walked over to the 1 WTC reflecting

pool where I joined Hayden and Steve. The three of us stood there silently. The scene of such an enormous trespass on my life—something that took me to the depths of hell—had become a place of peace. I looked down into the pool and then up to the sky. "Thank you, God. Thank you," I said, as a tear rolled down my cheek.

With that, I took Steve and Hayden's hands, and we walked from Ground Zero into our next adventure.

*

There is an invisible bond that ties all 9/11 survivors together. I often meet people who were in New York on that fateful day. Rarely, though, have I met anyone who was there, on the ground, in the same places I was—someone who shared and saw the same horrors. How ironic it was, then, that I met a member of the FDNY's Marine 1 Unit the afternoon before I left New York.

This firefighter showed us Fire Boat 343. Steel from the original 1 WTC was used to create parts of it, including the number 343—a number that is seared into the memory of all first responders. It signifies the number of firefighters who were killed on 9/11.

He told me he ran into 1 WTC after it was hit. I told him I was running out. He told me of all the sleepless nights, the nightmares, the drinking that happened after. I shared with him the same about me. He told me he married his wife after 9/11. I told him I married Steve soon after, too. He told me he had gotten help and now is okay. I told him how I was helped, too. He told me he has an eight-year-old son. I smiled and said, "So do I."

He and I were meant to meet before I left the city. We are

EPILOGUE

both examples of lives torn apart and then rebuilt, just like the new 1 WTC. We are both comfortable with the word *hero* now. We both go to work every day knowing that we make a difference. We sometimes laugh when we talk about the memories, and sometimes we cry. Our greatest hope is that people everywhere remember us and how we served on that day . . . and how we lost on that day, because WE WILL NEVER FORGET.

As the train pulled away from New York's Penn Station, I was filled with pride and a true feeling of being free. I was proud that I made the trip and proud of my process of forgiveness. I was proud of Steve for being a patient husband and a strong and caring father. I was proud of Hayden for asking the tough questions. I had closure, and now New York City is a special place that I look forward to visiting for years to come.

ACKNOWLEDGMENTS

ALMOST FIFTEEN YEARS have passed since that terrible, life-changing day. There were so many people who graciously opened their hearts and passed on their incredible wisdom and strength to me. I will be forever grateful.

First, I want to thank God. I know You have always been there despite my blindness. This book and the lessons I've learned would never have been if 9/11 did not happen. Thank You for trusting me with the scars.

To my mom: No matter what life threw at you, you always found a way to gain strength from it. Thank you for being my protector, my shoulder to cry on, my friend, and the person who gave me Harriet's name and number so I could get well.

To my husband, Steve—my Superman, the man who touched my heart: Thank you for not giving up on me, for not giving up on us.

To my son, Hayden: One day when you are older, you will read this and know how you helped keep your mom in check. Your laughter and bright smile reminds me of how precious life is. I love you with all my heart and soul.

To Harriett Yoselle: You saved my life. Your ability to heal knows no boundaries. I will be forever grateful.

To my grandparents, Nan and Papa Harry: I know you are

looking down from heaven. When things got tough, I could close my eyes and think of you as you wrapped me a warm hug. Your spirits live on in this book. Thank you for being "with me" through the process.

To my friend Artemis Limpert (artemislimpert.com): Thank you for "getting in my face" that day and making me realize what is most important in my life. Through the laughter and tears, you have taught me so many valuable lessons. Thank you for helping me break through barriers and honor my journey.

To Eyvonne and Dale Williams: Thank you for graciously taking me in at one of the toughest points in my life. Thank you for your amazing ability to heal, which set me back on the path to being well again. You both are true gifts to this world!

To Dr. Brown: Thank you for your encouragement, especially on the tough days. Thank you for helping me "see" my mission and stay connected with my faith. You have opened my eyes to the infinite wonders of what is possible.

To my very special sweetie pie in heaven, Solomon. Your spirit is always with me. You refused to lay down when you were gravely ill as a puppy, and you showed me what silent compassion was on that night when you saved my life. I saw it in your precious puppy dog eyes. We were meant to share part of our lives together. I know we will see each other again.

To the other two doctors in my life, Dr. Ben and Dr. K: Thank you for your encouraging words and for always being there to find solutions.

To my high school English teacher, Joy Adler: Thank you for giving me a C in writing. It helped me to dig deeper and become a more creative person, and it gave me the courage to write this book.

ACKNOWLEDGMENTS

To my amazing editor, Claudia: Although we met each other through another business, who knew we would be reintroduced and collaborate together? You have been a patient teacher. I so appreciate your guidance and input on this special project.

To Alecsey Boldeskul, the photographer who created a lifelong memory of our rescue that day: I will forever be grateful to you for stepping out amongst the chaos to preserve this moment in history.

To all my friends in the Dallas, Texas, area: What an adventure it has been! Ya'll have blessed my life beyond words. We have shared so much together—business meetings, months of travel, sleepless nights full of laughter at Success Camp, and all those crazy, fun houses we rented. But more than that, it is who you are that makes me want to be a better person in this world. I love you guys: Artemis Limpert, Don Broughton, Jordan Taylor, Gigi Coker, Stephanie Kirkpatrick, Catharine Dean, Diane Vessells, Ann and Tom Houghteling, Debra Evans, Dr. Mikey, Christine McGuire, Holly Bryan, and my incredibly bearded friend Jacob Burns.

To DaVinci and Lucy: You will never be able to read my book, but you provided me with warm shoulders to cry on and you licked away my tears on those bad days. You nudged my arm off the keyboard when it was time to play, and you kept me warm when the couch was my workspace. I love you guys.

Finally, to all those thought leaders, mentors, and teachers who helped bring me "into the light": The congruence with which you lead your lives is an inspiration. I have learned so much from you all: Brendon Burchard, Artemis Limpert, Tony Robbins, Robin Sharma, Ruben Gonzalez, Darren Hardy, and Gay Hendricks.

ABOUT THE AUTHOR

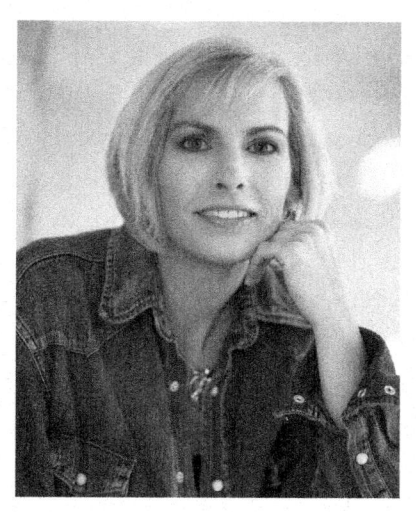

After graduating from the University of Maryland, College Park, and Howard University School of Law, Samantha Horwitz was accepted by the United States Secret Service. She was the only female in her graduating class to complete extensive training at the Federal Law Enforcement Training Center (FLETC) and the James J. Rowley Training Center (JJRTC) located just outside Washington, DC. She was assigned to the New York Field Office, Electronic Crimes Task Force, and in addition to investigative casework, she provided protection to several United States presidents, former presidents, first ladies, and many foreign dignitaries.

September 11, 2001, was a turning point in her life . . .

Sam was in the World Trade Center's North Tower when American Airlines Flight 11 struck it. After many difficult months, she made the heart-wrenching decision to leave the USSS due to the effects of PTSD (post-traumatic stress disorder).

After struggling with PTSD, alcoholism, and a suicide attempt, she found the help she needed and got well. She then pursued a career in the health and wellness industry as a franchise owner of a sports performance center in Rockville, Maryland, providing others with a place to get well and stay healthy.

After realizing that law enforcement was still "in her blood," Sam closed the sports performance center and returned to the law enforcement community in Montgomery County, Maryland, as a lieutenant assigned to the Executive Protection Detail. Her law enforcement career spanned twelve years, and she retired in 2012.

Sam is a successful entrepreneur, business owner, and speaker. She is a firearms instructor, and she runs Heroes 4 Healing, a unique outreach program for current and former first responders, law enforcement, and members of the U.S. military who are suffering from the effects of PTSD. Sam passes on her lessons of how she beat the odds and persevered through the darkest time in her life. By sharing her own personal struggle, she assists others to navigate their way back to wholeness and pursue their greatness!

Sam, her husband, Steve, her son, Hayden, and their two dogs, DaVinci and Lucy, reside in Rockwall, Texas.

To contact Sam about speaking at your next event, personal or media appearances, send an email to sam@courageaboveall.com. To connect with Sam on Facebook, visit www.facebook.com/courageaboveall.